MENTAL ILLNESS
AND
SOCIAL PROCESSES

Readers in Social Problems

Donald R. Cressey, consulting editor
UNIVERSITY OF CALIFORNIA,
SANTA BARBARA

MENTAL ILLNESS

AND

SOCIAL PROCESSES

THOMAS J. SCHEFF

EDITOR

HARPER & ROW

Publishers

NEW YORK, EVANSTON, AND LONDON

Library of Congress Catalog Card Number: 67-10802

CONTENTS

Introduction

THE ARTICLES in this reader represent recent thinking and research on a topic that might best be called the societal reaction to mental disorder. The theme that is common to most of the contributions is a concern with recurring patterns of behavior among individuals and organizations attempting to cope with persons who are defined as mentally ill. Perhaps at first glance this topic would seem to be excessively narrow. The reader might ask how it is that from the vast literature on mental illness the perspective of the societal reaction was chosen, since it represents only a small fraction of the total picture. This introductory essay is an attempt to answer this question, and to justify the choice of the societal reaction as a significant approach to the study of mental illness.

From the medical point of view it is traditional to divide the total field of mental illness, like any other disease, into four major areas: etiology, pathology, epidemiology, and therapy. Etiology is the study of causation; in the field of mental illness it remains one of the great puzzles in modern medicine. Pathology is the study of signs and symptoms that indicate the presence of disease. Conventionally in medicine, signs represent indications of disease that are observable to the physician; symptoms are the subjective reports of discomfort or difficulty made to the physician by the patient. Epidemiology is the study of the distribution of the disease in the entire population. From studies that include both the healthy and the sick, valuable clues concerning the causes of disease are often found. Finally, therapy concerns treatment and rehabilitation.

Social science has had rather little to offer in the first two

All footnotes appear in the Notes section, grouped by article, at the end of this book.

realms—etiology and pathology—which have been left largely to the investigations of psychiatrists and psychologists. The greatest contribution of social science has been in epidemiology. It is probably not an exaggeration to say that one of the chief sources of new insights into mental illness in recent years has been from the findings of medical epidemiologists and social scientists investigating the ecology and demography of mental illness. The work of Faris and Dunham, Hollingshead and Redlich, Pasamanick, Srole and his collaborators, and Leighton and his collaborators are some notable examples of this type of work.

The fourth and final medical approach to the problem of mental illness is that of therapy. The analogous area in social science is somewhat broader, including not only the description of psychiatric treatment and rehabilitation, but also the reaction of members of the community to mental illness: the study of the societal reaction. The largest group of studies in this area concerns the experience of patients in mental hospitals and clinics. There are also studies of community reactions to mental illness and education about mental illness, studies of decision-making about potential patients in the community, and surveys of attitudes toward mental illness. Examples of these studies and discussions of their implications for policy and theory constitute the subject matter of this book.

It is important that the reader understand that this book does not represent all of the contributions that social science has made to the study of mental disorder. It does present one major approach: the societal reaction. Another important approach in social science concerns epidemiology: the distribution of disease in entire populations. Since these two approaches complement one another, a knowledge of both is necessary to appreciate the concerns of current research in the social science of mental disorder.

It should also be noted that the study of the societal reaction is somewhat broader and more abstract than social epidemiology. By and large, epidemiological studies are conducted within the medical or psychiatric framework, accepting, without reservations, the various assumptions that are implicit in the medical model of mental illness. (The major exception to this statement is the study by Hollingshead and Redlich. Because their study of the handling of the mentally ill in New Haven goes far beyond mere counting of cases, it does raise questions about the medical model, and provides therefore, a link between the epidemiological and societal reaction approaches.) By and large, the researchers who have studied the societal reaction have tended not to accept the medical model, and to postulate models of mental illness that are different from the conventional medical or psychological ones. To illustrate this point, it is instructive to consider some aspects of popular conceptions of mental illness, the views which are typically held by laymen concerning mental disorder.

Popular conceptions of mental illness are often oversimplified to the point where it is difficult to communicate the importance of careful theoretical formulations. The stereotype of mental illness as being virtually always equivalent to the grossest and wildest insanity is still a significant component of public opinion even though the sophistication of the public, at least in verbal expressions, has probably been increasing. The comment of an 18th-century physician on insanity reveals the aura of bias and disinterest that still surrounds mental illness:

Defining madness as "A delirium without a fever," and admitting that this "was not a very accurate" definition, he stated: "There is no great occasion to be solicitous about the definition of a disease which everybody knows."[1]

The superciliousness of this remark, a bland assumption of simplicity, is a theme that recurs in popular perspectives on mental illness in United States history, and, in subtler forms, in current public opinion.

The theme of simplicity, and even more, the attitude of detachment that characterize popular conceptions of mental illness provide a clue for locating the phenomena within its social context. The casual assumption of simplicity is reminiscent of situations involving racial or class distinctions. The superordinate group often holds stereotypes about the members of the subordinate group: "everybody knows" that Negroes are inferior or that the lower classes are incapable of governing themselves. In order to understand the situation of the mentally ill, this discussion suggests that one could profit by comparing their position with that of other subordinate minorities. Psychological processes such as stereotyping, projection, and stigmatization, and social processes such as rejection, segregation, and isolation characterize, to some degree, the orientation of the in-group toward the outgroup, regardless of the basis of distinction. The recurring cycle of exposé, reform, and apathy in mental hospitals, the failure of mental health campaigns, and many other large-scale phenomena in the area of mental illness can be understood within the framework of the social processes connected with the formation of status distinctions. (Cf. "Normal Deviants," by Goffman, in this book.)

The conceptualization of mental illness in the literature of psychiatry, clinical psychology, and other professional disciplines is obviously much more refined than that of the public. Nevertheless, there are consistent biases in this literature that can be qualified by social science perspectives. One such bias is the tendency to present only the most extreme cases of aberrant behavior in the clinical literature. This is a problem that occurs not only in psychiatry but in all science: for purposes of clarity, analytic categories are illustrated by polar cases. In the field of mental illness, however, the tendency to use extreme examples for analytic clarity reinforces the popular stereotype of the extremeness of mental illness, and serves also to reify behavioral classifications (such as paranoid behavior, depression) into concrete disease entities.

To be sure, it is necessary to make detailed observations of the behavior associated with mental illness. For this reason, clinical description of psychiatric symptoms is a prerequisite for any kind of analysis. The articles in this reader, many of them critical of contemporary psychiatric theory and classifications, nevertheless assume and depend upon the reader's familiarity with conventional psychiatric classifications, such as mania, schizophrenia, depression, and the various psychoneuroses, such as anxiety states, conversion hysteria, and so on. The reader who is not acquainted with psychiatric classifications should consult any of the standard textbooks in psychiatry or abnormal psychology.

It is equally true, however, that most clinical description does not convey the many kinds of ambiguity that are involved in psychiatric symptoms. The following textbook description of manic behavior will be used to illustrate some of the difficulties connected with using the clinical literature.

A thirty-five-year-old biochemist was brought to the clinic by his frightened wife. To his psychiatrist the patient explained, "I discovered that I had been drifting, broke the bonds and suddenly found myself doing things and doing them by telegraph. I was dead tired, and decided to go on a vacation; but even there it wasn't long before I was sending more telegrams. I got into high gear and started to buzz. Then a gentle hint from a friend took effect and I decided to come here and see if the changes in my personality were real." He entered the ward in high spirits, went about greeting the patients, insisted that the place was "swell," and made quick puns on the names of doctors to whom he was introduced. Meanwhile his wife said she was "scared to death." "His friends used to call him 'Crazy Charley,'" she said, "but I haven't seen this streak in him for years."

When his wife had left, the patient soon demonstrated what he meant by "high gear." He bounded down the hall, threw his medication on the floor, leaped on a window ledge and dared any one to get him down. When he was put in a room alone where he could be free, he promptly dismantled the bed, pounded on the walls, yelled and sang. He made a sudden sally into the hall and did a kind of hula-hula dance before he could be returned to his room. His shouting continued throughout the night and betrayed in its content the ambivalent attitudes which the patient maintained toward his hospitalization: "What the hell kind of place is this? A swell place? I'm not staying here. I'm having a hell of a good time. Oh, I'm so happy. I have to get going. My gray suit please, my gray coat please, my gray socks, all gray on their way, going to be gay, I'm going out as fast as I came in, only faster. I'm happier than I have ever been in my life. I'm 100 per cent better than normal."

The following morning, after almost no sleep, the patient was more noisy and energetic than ever. He smashed the overhead light with his shoes and ripped off the window guard. He tore up several hospital gowns, draped himself in a loin cloth made of their fragments, said he was Tarzan, and gave wild jungle cries to prove it. "I've tasted tiger's blood!" he roared. "I'm a success and I'm the man for my boss's job. I've made a killing and this time I will keep on going." He made amorous remarks to the nurses, accused them of flirting with him, and announced loudly, "At the present time I am not married; but my body is not for sale, regardless of the price."[2]

This excerpt clearly illustrates the chief characteristics of behavior that psychiatrists diagnose as manic: elation, flight of ideas, and hyperactivity. The case is misleading, however, in that in the typical case in which a diagnosis of mania is made, the indications are much more confused and unclear. Typically one or more of the following kinds of ambiguity might occur: the alleged symptoms are not so extreme and perhaps have some grounds, as for elation, for example. Moreover, the amount of information at the disposal of the diagnostician may be extremely limited and of uncertain reliability: garbled accounts of alleged incidents by hostile or confused family members are frequently the chief source of information. Often it would seem that the greater the amount of information about the symptoms, and the higher its quality, the less extreme and more understandable the "symptom" becomes. Frequently there is confusion because of conflicts between different accounts of the symptoms: the family may have one version, the patient another, and the diagnostician's own observations may suggest still another. Many of the patients seen by clinicians have been forced or tricked into the hospital; the clinician must unravel the "illness" from the reactions of the patient to coercion and/or duplicity. A further source of ambiguity is found in the tendency to medicate psychiatric patients first and ask questions later. The examining physician may have to decide, for example, to what extent the quiescence or even stupor of a new admittance is the result of earlier treatment.

A particularly central feature of the handling of the mentally ill in our society concerns the grounds upon which psychiatric treatment is sought. Because the textbook presentations of symptoms of mental patients tend to be unambiguous, the inference is usually made that the symptoms are the causes of the patient's difficulties, and particularly, the causes for the patient's seeking of psychiatric attention. Recent studies of the social processes involved in getting to a psychiatrist suggest, however, that economic, psychological, and social contingencies may be as important as, or more important than, the patient's symptoms.

A case observed by the author in the male admissions wards of an English mental hospital will illustrate the importance of contingencies in admission.

Charles Plumber was an 18-year-old student at Chesley Manor, a state school for "difficult" children through high school. The patient's father drove him 100 miles to see the doctor. The nursing aide had talked to him at the school a month or so earlier. He was virtually incoherent at that time also—"he couldn't be handled at home and wouldn't listen to his parents." One "extreme, furniture-smashing incident" was handled in courts, 3 and ½ years earlier.

The patient was a short, slight, red-haired male with sparse, scraggly facial hair which was not quite a beard. He had a suspicious and somewhat secretive manner. He laughed often—bitter little laughs, as if to himself. He carried one shoulder slightly higher than the other, and had a somewhat hunched posture. Charles' father commented, "He was getting on wonderfully well, [at the school] but three months ago, he went out of control, became uncommunicative. He refused to be gated [restricted to grounds]. Charles stole books from the local book stores; was found by the police in a phone booth at 5 A.M.; he locked himself in a public lavatory for 4 and ½ hours, then stated that he was there only 15 minutes. He seems to have lost track of time."

"He wanted to get a job, but was discouraged on recommendations from Mr. Lywood [principal of school]. He has deteriorated since that time. He forged his birth certificate to get a job." The father elaborates, explaining why Charles wasn't told he was being brought to a mental hospital. "I don't want to dump him here, but I don't see how I can bring him back to Chesley Manor, or take him home. I know this is hard, but can you help him?"

There was a one-hour interview with Charles, by myself, a female aide, a psychiatrist and the male "charge".

AUTHOR: Do you work on any hobbies at school?
PATIENT: "I is D. I is attitude; D is determination. I is the opposite of D.
A: Is there anything you are particularly interested in?
P: Commercialization *vs.* wear and tear.
A: What is commercialization?
P: It's the car bodies. You drill holes in the car bodies to see if they will come through. Are you doing any research here on cars?
DOCTOR: No, we don't do any work on cars.
P: I am interested in electronics, the electronics of cars. It's got to be tested over and over again.

After some thirty minutes, in which Charles responded irrelevantly and incoherently to at least one hundred questions, the doctor asked:

DR.: Would you like to stay here with us for a while? We could probably help you, and you could find some pals here on the ward, and do some of the things that you like to do.
P: No. This place frightens me. I want to go back to school.

Thus after a half hour of confusion, Charles responded rapidly and succinctly to the fundamental question of the whole interview—did he want to be hospitalized—with a clear and emphatic no.

The father was a mild, bland, lower-middle class Englishman, quite deferential toward the staff. I asked him, after the interview, "Do you ever have any trouble understanding what your son is saying?"

FATHER: "Oh, yes. You mean that jargon. I don't know where he gets it from. He certainly didn't learn it at home."

The doctor asked the father if he wished to have the boy committed, since it was obvious that Charles would not enter informally [in the English system, roughly equivalent to voluntary hospitalization.] "No, I told him we were just going to see a doctor. That's how I got him to come. If I tricked him now, I would betray whatever trust there is left between us."

The doctor agreed, and suggested that he phone the headmaster and suggest that Charles be taken back on trial. The doctor told the headmaster that if there were any difficulties, he should call the hospital, and he would handle things from there. The headmaster agreed. Charles was taken back to school, and a month later, we still hadn't heard from him.

Two important points should be noted about this case. First, it was fairly clear that Charles has been exhibiting a pattern of psychiatric symptoms over a period of years. These include autism, mutism, irrelevance, and incoherence of speech, or "word salads." Yet, the behavior that was effective in bringing him to psychiatric attention was not the symptoms but the deviant behavior that caused difficulty for the school and his parents.

Secondly, the "patient" was not hospitalized, even though the psychiatrist and all other staff members present viewed the patient's behavior as obviously psychotic—a "textbook case." The failure to hospitalize Charles Plumber was particularly striking to the author, because it occurred after he had viewed a series of admission interviews in which much milder and more ambiguous "symptoms" had been the grounds for admission. In the series of admissions observed, it was clear that except in the rare, extreme cases (4 out of the 50) it was not the symptoms of mental illness that were effective in deciding the "patient's" fate, but other contingencies. In the case described above, the "patient" exhibited clear and unambiguous psychiatric symptoms: speech distortions of the type usually ascribed to schizophrenics. Yet these symptoms were decisive with neither the father nor the psychiatrist. The father's reaction was bland and diffuse

("Oh, you mean that jargon. I don't know where he gets it from, he certainly didn't learn it at home.") The psychiatrist obviously viewed the patient as mentally ill, but honored the father's decision not to hospitalize. In this case, as well as in others described in the literature, it was clear that recognition and treatment of mental illness depended on a complex chain of circumstances in which psychiatric symptoms were at best only a small part.

The recognition that the medical point of view, when applied to mental illness, systematically obscures important psychological and social processes has been developed by a number of psychiatrists and social scientists. Harry Stack Sullivan, a prominent American psychiatrist, formulated a theory in which mental illness was viewed less as an illness than as a disturbance of interpersonal relations.[3] More recently, Thomas Szasz, another psychiatrist, has argued that mental illness is a myth, and that psychiatric "symptoms" should be interpreted within a "game-playing" point of view.[4] The sociologists Lemert and Goffman have suggested sociological frames of reference for the understanding of mental illness.[5] A recent collection of articles makes readily available a wide variety of criticisms of, and departures from, the application of the medical model to mental illness.[6]

The articles in this reader do not attempt to replace the medical model with a single psychological or sociological model of "mental illness," but approach the problem from widely different perspectives. A unifying theme in these articles is one of methodology rather than theory. The authors seek what might be described as an anthropological perspective: to avoid the explicit and implicit assumptions that members of the society make about mental illness, they approach the topic as outsiders. This approach is known in anthropology as the study of "folk medicine": it seeks to describe the behavior of members of a society with respect to illness without necessarily sharing the assumptions that are made in that society about illness.

It is clear that different social groups not only have different rates of illness, but to some extent, different kinds of illness. Thus the disease entity which the French refer to as a "foie" (liver) is widely recognized and treated in France, but not in the United States. "Listo," an illness caused by fright, and "empacho," or stomach disorder, are found in Mexico, and among Mexican-Americans in the United States, but not elsewhere.[7] Apparently there are a wide variety of diseases that are culturally unique. The phenomena of death through hexing or bone-pointing has been described by numerous anthropologists. These phenomena can be studied best as "folk medicine": the researcher can describe the patterns of symptoms, treatments, outcomes, and beliefs held by the patients and medicine men, in an objective manner, without himself necessarily subscribing to these beliefs.

The approach of "folk medicine," applied to the study of mental illness, implies that the investigator can describe the patterns of behavior and beliefs with regard to mental illness without necessarily accepting (or rejecting) them himself. The most important assumption about mental illness in Western society is that it *is an illness*, and should be considered and treated as an illness. The approach suggested here would treat this assumption as an important part of the field of study, as a folk belief, about which the investigator seeks to remain impartial.

To illustrate some of the implications of this approach, let us consider some alternative interpretations of a single case. The following was reported in *The Milwaukee Journal*. It was accompanied by a picture of Mrs. _____, showing a serene and benign middle-aged matron, posing before some religious art in her house.

NECEDAH WOMAN STILL HAS "VISIONS"
Mrs. _____ Lives Quietly on Farm,
Says Virgin Mary's Visits Continue.

Mrs. _____ says she still talks with the Virgin Mary. The Catholic church has discounted her visions. Some who believed in them once no longer do. Most never believed.

But Mrs. _____ doesn't care. She has faith that someday her band of followers will become a legion. The scoffing, the disbelief, the ridicule are all part of her mission, the farm woman believes.

For 12 years she has remained true in her mind to the promises she says she made to carry out the mission of Mary's message to the people: "Pray, pray. . . . for only prayers will save the destruction of this world."

BELIEVERS ARE EXPECTED

In the next four days, some hundreds of believers are expected to make the trip to the farm in a secluded, wooded area two miles from this Juneau County community. The Virgin is supposed to have appeared before Mrs. _____ on those same four dates in 1950.

The followers will listen to the 52-year-old woman tell of the Virgin's appearances and will pray at a new outdoor shrine named in honor of St. Anne, mother of Mary.

On these anniversary days, Mrs. _____ says, the apparition of the Virgin Mary reappears, as Mary promised.

100,000 WERE THERE

Once, on Aug. 15, 1950, about 100,000 persons made the pilgrimage to the farm, coming from all over the country.

The farm wife's story began the night of Nov. 12, 1949. She says she was awakened and saw a vision—the Virgin Mary. The next visit was on Good Friday, April 7, 1950, when the Virgin appeared as a strange glow around the figure on her crucifix, Mrs. _____ said.

This time the Virgin Mary spoke:

"Yes, pray my child . . . your cross is heavy to bear, but the people all over the world are facing a heavier cross and sorrow with the enemy of God unless we pray, pray hard with all our hearts devotedly."

DATES ANNOUNCED

There were six other visits, the dates of which had all been announced on Mary's visit on May 28, 1950, Mrs. _____ said.

In a troubled world, with war raging in Korea, the Virgin's messages as transmitted through Mrs. _____ were hopefully picked up by many.

The climax came on Aug. 15. Only Mrs. _____ among the 100,000 saw the vision that day. In the farm wife's words, recorded that day:

"The Blessed Mother appeared to me . . . at 12 o'clock noon. There was a blue mist south of the four ash trees as I opened the kitchen door to walk out. The blue mist comes through the tips of the trees and forms into Our Lady. She smiled as I approached."

DRESSED IN WHITE

"At the other time, Our Mother was dressed in blue. Today she was in white, a real dazzling white, so brilliant and radiant. All her garments were white. Her veil was a very thin material.

"On her head she had a wreath of small, pink roses. She had the same golden cord around her neck with a globe of the world and the tassel. She again stood on a pillow or cloud with large pink roses on it. She was barefooted and held the same large rosary. She smiled as I approached her and looked over the crowd smiling."

Mrs. _____ then addressed the crowd, concluding: "We have no time to lose. We must carry out our program now—at once—for prayer only will save us."

APPEARS DURING LENT

Mrs. _____ said recently that the Virgin Mary's appearances were not daily but were on the anniversary dates and on the Fridays during

Lent and Advent. Mrs. _____ said she suffered "the passion of our Lord" on those Fridays.

She said it was "pretty hard to explain. It's a different type of suffering that one can only feel in one's own system in witnessing the passions of our Lord." Most of the pains occur between the hours of noon and 3 P.M., she said.

A former Milwaukeean, Miss _____ takes down messages Mrs. _____ transmits. They are mimeographed and mailed to her followers in every state but Hawaii, and to some in foreign countries.

Another companion of the farm woman is Miss _____, a woman in her sixties who has been with Mrs. _____ since the visions began.

DESCRIBES JESUS

"On Holy Thursday," Miss _____ said, "the suffering begins at 9 P.M. and continues until midnight. _____ witnesses the Lord and the Holy Mother during the Last Supper and the first mass."

Asked for a description of Jesus as she sees Him, Mrs. _____ referred to a painting on the dining room wall.

"This picture makes Him look very handsome. . . . As I see him, He is more muscular and I see Him with blue eyes, not brown eyes. He has a beard and is a well built man with lighter hair and is more muscular than shown here."

Mrs. _____ said she couldn't understand conversation between Jesus and the apostles: "You see, they don't talk our language."

WARNS ABOUT MORALITY

She said she had "an area of a 30-mile radius that I suffer for, which would include Tomah, Mauston and as far as Wisconsin Dells. The warnings are all there to clean out your newsstands, dens, your taverns and things."

"The holy mother doesn't say anything against the Protestants," Mrs. _____ said in answer to a question. "A good many Protestants are better Christians than some Catholics."

Mrs. _____ was born in Philadelphia, the second of six children of Mr. and Mrs. _____, who were born in Rumania. The family had lived in Ohio, then moved to Pleasant Prairie (Kenosha county) Wis., in 1914. Mrs. _____ had no church affiliation but attended Methodist Sunday school.

In 1934, she married her husband and became a Catholic. He died in 1960.

BUILT A NEW HOME

The couple moved around to Texas, Missouri and finally to Hurley, Wis., in 1938. In 1942, they moved to Juneau county and to the present 142 acre farm in 1944.

Fire destroyed their old house in 1959, but they built a new, cement block house near by.

There are still two teenage children at home, and Mrs. _____ is concerned for their welfare.

"I don't care about myself. I can take it—the persecution. But it's the children that get hurt."

She dislikes publicity and says the newspaper stories have "sensationalized" her story.

SHE CLAIMS SUPPORT

However, many people wrote testimonials—to counteract newspaper stories—telling that they, too, saw the Virgin Mary appear on Aug. 15, Oct. 7, 1950.

"The sun spun in the sky!" many people wrote her, Mrs. _____ said.

Bishop John P. Treacy of La Crosse has denounced the visions as false and Mrs. _____ says she thinks the church would rather forget about the whole thing.

She still attends mass in Necedah, however, and says that the church's attitude toward her visions is just part of the cross she has to bear.[8]

The text makes clear that one interpretation that has been made of Mrs. _____'s behavior is in a religious context. According to the interpretation of her followers, and Mrs. _____ herself, her visions were of supernatural origin. From this point of view, the source of the messages Mrs. _____ hears is the Virgin Mary. Apparently a sizeable group of persons shared this interpretation at one time, and some still retain their belief.

A second interpretation, perhaps the majority point of view, is that the sources of Mrs. _____'s visions are not supernatural, but are a product of disease. From this point of view, the medical point of view, the visions and messages are visual and auditory hallucinations, and most of her religious beliefs are delusions. These manifestations are not products of supernatural intervention in human affairs, but the intrusions of disease.

Although the religious and medical interpretations of Mrs. _____'s behavior obviously are fundamentally different, they are similar in that they both posit a cause and course of behavior that lie outside of human experience: in the religious perspective, divine intervention, and from the medical point of view, the onslaught of disease. But divine intervention and disease are equally exterior and accidental to the flow of human affairs. These viewpoints are similar also in that there is little scientifically acceptable evidence supporting the appearance of divine beings on earth, or for the cause

and course of functional mental illnesses, such as schizophrenia.

For the social scientist, however, the symptoms of mental
illness have human meaning and human consequences regardless of their origins. Whether "psychiatric symptoms"
originate in supernatural occurrences, disease, stress, or voli-
tional acts, these behaviors can be viewed in the context of
the human conditions in which they occur, the patterns of
reactions to the behavior by others, and the typical outcomes
of the behavior for the individual and his community. Thus
the approach of "folk medicine" does not depend on theological or medical arguments about the initial causes of symptomatic behavior, but can proceed to describe the behavior, the
conditions for its recognition, treatment, and termination,
and the beliefs of the mentally ill and those reacting to them.

The agnostic stance of the social scientist toward mental
illness frees him from the clinical preoccupation with the
single patient, and enables him to point out some of the
larger social issues that are connected with mental illness.
To the extent that the medical point of view toward aberrant
behavior has become institutionalized, certain internal contradictions have appeared between medical institutions and
other institutions in Western society. The current view accepted in our society that "mental illness is just like any
other illness" has created discrepancies between medical and
legal institutions, for example. These contradictions occur
in a number of areas, but three illustrations will suffice in
connection with hospitalization, divorce, and criminal justice.

Perhaps the clearest contradiction in our current medical
institutions is the phenomena of having mental hospitals in
which the majority of patients receive no treatment. According to the report of the Joint Commission on Mental Health
and Illness:

It is natural of course that we should wish to emphasize gains as a
buttress to an attitude of constructive hope as source of renewed en-
ergy. One thing recent progress has done is to show that tangible
changes can be produced through increased governmental initiative,
public attention, pressure and support, thus putting to rout the attitude
of cynicism and futility, that has been connected with the custodial
care of the mentally ill for so long.

But if we are to be wholly honest with ourselves and with the public, then we must view the mental health problem in terms of the unmet need, those who are untreated and inadequately cared for . . . *the information we have leads us to believe that more than ½ of the patients in most state hospitals receive no active treatment of any kind designed to improve their mental condition.* This applies to most of the patients on "continued treatment" wards, a term actually meaning "discontinued treatment," the supposition being that the patient's illness has progressed from an acute to a chronic stage.[9]

The cycle of exposé, reform, and apathy which has characterized the treatment of the mentally ill in the United States for over a hundred years, finds us still with hospitals that are more like prisons than hospitals.

A second contradiction occurs in those states in which chronic mental illness is grounds for divorce. The marriage vows explicitly state that the marriage contract is to be honored in "sickness and in health." Physical sickness, no matter how chronic or incurable, is not grounds for divorce, but mental illness is. The discrepancy between the institution of mental illness, and physical illness, and the legal institution of divorce is apparent in this case.

A final contradiction that will be discussed lies in the question of criminal responsibility. The use of mental illness to excuse responsibility for committing a crime has given rise to extensive controversy between the legal and the medical professions. This controversy is ably discussed in a wide variety of settings, and will not be further elaborated here. There are a large number of questions relating to responsibility that arise in contexts other than criminal trials, which have not been as well covered. The following letter to the editor of a newspaper, and the editor's reply, illustrate one facet of this issue.

SAYS WE HARASSED WEATHERLY
By Rev. Max Gaebler, Minister,
First Unitarian Society of Madison

It is disturbing to note how often newspapers which give overt encouragement to the mental health movement remain insensitive to the extent to which their own manner of handling the news affects the goals of that movement. So it happens that the very paper which gives coverage to a mental health workshop does untold damage to individuals through its failure to recognize and to deal compassionately with emotional disturbance.

It is because of this concern that your editorial of July 26 regarding Bruce Weatherly's death now moves me to record thoughts which I should have preferred to leave unspoken. Your effort to undo Mr. Weatherly's appointment as Madison's Chief of Police, thwarted in the courts, was early converted into an unwavering campaign of harassment against Mr. Weatherly himself.

Under this unremitting pressure his evident emotional problems were aggravated until it had become apparent to virtually everyone that he could no longer properly discharge his duties. Nonetheless, blind to the fact that he was a sick man, blind to the pain such a situation must under the best of circumstances have caused his family, and utterly blind to the extent to which your own campaign of harassment might have contributed to Mr. Weatherly's condition, you exposed him to the ultimate indignities in the course of those events which led to his dismissal.

That he and his family were able to survive those events at all is remarkable. But it is now evident that the damage was irreparable, and the final scene in the tragic history of Bruce Weatherly has now been enacted. The truly tragic character of that story and your unenviable role in it might have been allowed to remain unstated had you had at least the final decency to refrain from further comment.

Unhappily you have seen fit to reiterate the most unsavory aspects of Mr. Weatherly's career, and you conclude by congratulating yourself for having been right from the first. It is this unwarranted conclusion which compels me to write this word of protest. The fact is that Mr. Weatherly's inadequacies were in no way related to his having come from out of the state; Wisconsin natives are as liable to mental and emotional illness as those from Texas.

And the fact also is that those inadequacies, in Mr. Weatherly's case, might well have been arrested and his very real talents given proper scope, or failing that, genuine rehabilitation might have been possible even after his dismissal from his position here, had your newspaper shown even a modicum of human sympathy and understanding in your relationship with him.

That is now past, and the tragedy is fulfilled. We can only hope that out of the present darkness some new hope may kindle for Mrs. Weatherly and her family. And we can seek forgiveness for her, for her late husband, for you and for us all.

OUR REPLY

(Editor's Note—The Capital Times brought action in court to block the Weatherly appointment relying on Sec. 66.11 (1) of the then Wisconsin statute providing: "No person shall be appointed deputy sheriff or police officer of any county or city unless he is a citizen of the United States and shall have resided in this state continuously for one year immediately preceding." Our position was upheld by Circuit Judge Kenneth White, a long time political foe of The Capital Times who recognized that the law involved was written to strengthen the morale of public officials by helping to assure promotion from within the ranks.

The State Supreme Court ruled that a police chief was not a "police officer." While that may make it the law it doesn't make it good sense. This was the same court that ruled McCarthy had done everything he was accused of doing but refused to discipline him.

The drinking habits, which were finally to be Weatherly's undoing, manifested themselves soon after he took over his job. We did not regard this as proper activity for a man in charge of enforcing the laws of this City, particularly the laws governing liquor traffic. Mr. Gaebler may be well enough trained or gifted in psychoanalysis to be able to say that his trouble was "emotional problems." Unfortunately we are not. We saw it as a chief law enforcement officer spending too much time drinking in taverns and thereby weakening law enforcement in Madison.

It was not easy to make a case against Weatherly. He had powerful friends defending him, including one of the daily papers in Madison. The extent to which they would go to defend him was illustrated by the fact that one member of the Police and Fire Commission, Marshal Browne, voted to retain him even after his final escapade when he destroyed a police car after an afternoon and evening of heavy drinking.

The Capital Times does not regard it as a duty of a newspaper to psychoanalyze people in public life. We are not equipped to do so and we would not even if we were. It is a tough enough job to keep tabs on those who are violating the public trust they assume when they take public office.

This is particularly true where the liquor traffic is concerned. Its influence penetrates deeply into all levels of government, but nowhere more seriously than in the state legislature where its control is unquestioned by any informed observer.

In fighting this evil in state government we have had to injure some officeholders with tender sensitivities, probably "emotional problems," if one can judge from the drinking parties that go on in the night clubs and hotel rooms around the Square. If we didn't do it the beer cans and whiskey bottles would be raining out of the hotel windows in downtown Madison.

We would like a little help from some of the spiritual leaders of the community, such as Mr. Gaebler, in trying to keep this evil in bounds. But somehow they always seem to be occupied elsewhere, probably immersed in psychoanalytical work.[10]

The medical institution of mental illness introduces a wholly new vocabulary of motive and rhetoric of responsibility into social and political issues. The focus of the mental health clinician on the isolated single case tends to obscure such issues. Social science perspectives such as those in these articles, although they do not always adequately handle the fine details of the picture, do make room for, and encourage the recognition of the functions and contradictions in mental illness, for the patient, the community, and the larger society. In this and other ways, social science perspectives may come to complement, but not replace, clinical views.

The first three sections of this reader concern the sequence of social-psychological events in the handling of mental illness. The first section deals with the problem of lay classifications of behavior as normal or abnormal: the nature of the categories and stereotypes that are called into play in the "recognition" of mental illness. The second section is devoted to the judgmental processes that occur after a "diagnosis" of suspected mental illness has been made. The decision-makers may be community elders, lawyers, judges, physicians, or psychiatrists. The third section concerns social and psychological processes that are involved in psychiatric treatment after the diagnosis has been confirmed and acted upon. The final section treats some of the conceptual and policy issues that arise when the medical model is replaced by a more inclusive perspective. It is hoped that the clash of these divergent points of view will lead to more adequate policy and research programs in the future.

PART I

"Recognition" of Mental Illness—The Definitional Process

In the first article in this section, David Mechanic provides an over-all viewpoint of the significance of social definitions of mental illness. He argues that contrary to the popular view (that social definitions are unimportant because only the opinion of the psychiatrist is crucial), social definitions predominate in the channeling of mentally ill persons into, or away from, psychiatric treatment. Mechanic goes on to discuss some of the contingencies which determine whether or not nonconforming behavior is defined as evidence of mental illness.

In the second article, Yarrow, Schwartz, Murphy, and Deasy present case material which illustrates Mechanic's points. This article describes the initial reactions of 33 wives to their husbands' psychiatric symptoms. It should be noted that this group of cases was selected through admissions to a psychiatric facility. The process described, therefore, represents only cases in which the husbands "settled down" to a psychiatric illness. Because we have very little evidence on the outcomes of a randomly selected group of persons exhibiting psychiatric symptoms in the community, the reader should resist the temptation to conclude that psychiatric symptoms are reliable signs that sustained mental illness will occur. Indeed, the extremely high prevalence of psychiatric symptoms reported in community psychiatric surveys strongly suggests the opposite: most psychiatric symptoms are "denied" in the community (as the wives initially denied their husbands' symptoms in the present article), and do not go on to become sustained mental illness.

The problem of the prognostic value of psychiatric signs (observable behavior) and symptoms (subjective reports) is a crucial one in current psychiatry. Proponents of preventive psychiatry argue that it is necessary to "reach out" into the community, find and treat mental illness before it becomes untreatable. Proponents of "containment" argue that "reaching out" would be a mistake: psychiatrists, according to this *point of view, should avoid interfering with the natural psychological and community processes that handle deviance. In the majority of cases, they argue, the person and/or the community will find some way of coping with the difficulty, and the problems associated with psychiatric "labeling" will be side-stepped.*

If, as Mechanic argues, the process of defining mental illness is of fundamental significance, we need to know how people go about recognizing mental illness. The next two articles in this section supply information about popular stereotypes of mental illness. Nunnally's article reports the results from an extensive survey of stereotypes of mental illness in the mass media. Phillips' article presents the findings from an ingenious study of reactions to psychiatric symptoms under conditions where a psychiatric label had, and had not, been applied. This study demonstrates very convincingly the effects of "denial" and "labeling" on the "recognition" of mental illness. In the final paper in this section, Grey gives an autobiographical account of childhood stereotypes and experience with a mental patient that illustrates some of the definitional processes described in the other papers.

Some Factors in Identifying and Defining Mental Illness

The procedures through which persons in need of psychiatric treatment are identified and treated are frequently unclear. On some occasions persons exhibiting relatively mild symptoms are identified as psychiatric problems and appear for treatment, while persons with more serious psychiatric symptoms go unrecognized and untreated.

Yet the routes taken by patients who are brought to or appear at the hospital, clinic, or office of the private psychiatrist, provide the sociologist with an opportunity to illuminate the processes of patient selection and treatment.

A number of studies along these lines have contributed richly to our understanding of these processes.[1] These studies have pointed to the varying definitions of illness that are made at various locations in the social structure.[2] For example, the patient may view his own illness in terms of his feeling state; his employer might evaluate his symptoms in

From *Mental Hygiene* 46 (January, 1962) 66–74. Reprinted by permission of the author and the publisher.

Dr. Mechanic is Assistant Professor, Department of Sociology, The University of Wisconsin, Madison, Wis. This is a revised version of a paper presented at the Annual Meeting of the American Sociological Association in New York City in August, 1960. The impressions reported here stem, in part, from exploratory interviews and observations at two California hospitals. These observations were carried out with the assistance of Research Grant MF–8516 of the National Institute of Mental Health.

terms of his apparent deviation from group requirements; and his family may adjudge him "ill" on the basis of the attitude he professes or his situational behavior.

Yet definitions *are* made; patients *do* appear for treatment —although at times by rather devious routes—and psychiatric aid *is* administered. It is the major purpose of this paper to consider some of the definitions that are made, the conflicts that occur, the manner in which resolutions are attempted, and the effects of the definitional process on the eventual decisions as to who receives treatment.

In essence, I will draw a descriptive model of the definitional processes by which persons within a community are adjudged "mentally ill" by family, friends, community authorities and even by themselves, based on observations made at admission wards in two California mental hospitals and other reported research results.

The early definitions of mental illness, especially in middle-class populations, are likely to take place in the groups within which the person primarily operates; evaluations are made by family, fellow employees, friends, and employers. If symptoms appear and are not recognized as such by members of the individual's more primary groups, it is unlikely that he will become accessible to psychiatric personnel unless his symptoms become visible, and disturbing enough to lead to his commitment to some treatment center by external authorities.

On other occasions, it is the person himself, who, in comparing his feelings and behavior with how he thinks others feel and behave or with how he has felt and behaved in the past, defines himself as ill and seeks what he regards as competent help.

Finally, when patients appear for psychiatric treatment, either on their own volition or under pressure of significant others, the physician evaluates the symptoms and then comes to some decision about the "illness." These various evaluations by the person himself, by his social group, by community agencies, and by psychiatric experts may be more or less consistent. However, discrepancies often occur, and when they arise, adequate solutions for resolving these differences are not always readily available.

Problems of definition arise, in part, because all behaviors occur within specific group contexts, and the frames of reference of the evaluators are not always comparable. Also, since the evaluators may be located at different foci of interaction with the person, the behavior they see may differ significantly.

The behaviors defined as symptoms of "illness" may be as much characteristic of some particular situation or group setting as they are enduring attributes of persons. For example, even with purely physiological symptoms, social definitions are applied which have important consequences for the patient and the course of his illness. The symptom may be defined as a sign of "illness" and receive the usual considerations of the sick role, or it may be viewed as an unjustifiable attempt to seek relief from legitimate expectations. It may be evaluated as a symbol of high prestige and community status (as a battle wound) or it may be seen as a consequence of promiscuous and shameful activities (as might be the case with venereal disease). The symptom, in sum, may be worthy of group consideration, sympathy and support, or it may be punished, criticized, or ignored.

Persons with intangible neurotic symptoms which might be interpreted as signs of weakness and excessive self-concern are reacted to quite differently from, for example, persons who have difficulties during such stressful situations as bereavement.

Although seemingly obvious, it is important to state that what may be viewed as deviant in one social group may be tolerated in another, and rewarded in still other groups. How group members view a particular behavior is likely to influence both the frequency with which it occurs and the extent to which it is exhibited. In other words, all groups exercise considerable control over their members.

"Mental illness" and other forms of deviancy become visible when persons in the participant's group recognize his inability and reluctance to make the proper responses in his network of interpersonal relations. How a particular deviant behavior is to be evaluated depends largely on the frame of reference the evaluators assume. Whether a deviant act is seen as evidence of "crime," "corruption," "illness," and so

on, will be contingent on the criteria with which the evaluator operates and how he applies them.

It is hypothesized that the evaluator attempts to understand
the motivation of the actor. In the language of Mead, he
assumes the role of the other and attempts to empathize. If
the empathy process is successful, the evaluator is likely to
feel that he has some basis for labeling the deviant act as
"delinquency," "undependability," or whatever.[3] It is primarily in those cases where the evaluator feels at a loss in
adequately empathizing with the actor and where he finds it
difficult to understand what attributed to the response that
the behavior is more likely to be labeled "queer," "strange,"
"odd," or "sick."

There are behaviors, however, where the distinction is
unclear; where, for example, an understandable crime is
committed, but the expressed motive makes little sense; it
thus becomes difficult to decide whether the actor is a
"criminal," a potential "mental patient," or both.[4] In general,
however, mental illness is regarded usually as a residual
category for deviant behavior having no clearly specified
label.

Of course the physician trained in the treatment of the
mentally ill, applies different criteria to behavior than does
the layman. The criteria he applies to deviant behavior are
more closely related to the theory of pathology he holds than
to his own ability or inability to take the role of the other.
The criteria he holds, however, are at times indefinite and
the physician who practices in large treatment centers often
must assume the illness of the patient who appears before
him and then proceed to prescribe treatment. Both the
abstract nature of the physician's theories and the time
limitations imposed upon him by the institutional structure
of which he is a part make it impossible for him to make a
rapid study of the patient's illness or even to ascertain if
illness, in fact, exists. Instead, it becomes necessary for him
to assume the illness of the patient and to apply some label
to the alleged if not recognizable symptoms. The consequences are that the basic decision about illness usually
occurs prior to the patient's admission to the hospital and
this decision is more or less made by nonprofessional mem-

bers of the community. It therefore becomes a matter of considerable interest to understand how these nonprofessional members of the community define "mental illness."

Before moving on to discuss the variables affecting community definitions of "mental illness," it is important to emphasize in more detail the preceding point: that the basic decision about illness is usually made by community members and *not professional personnel*. Although the very "sick" are usually found in mental hospitals, there are occasions when very "sick" persons go unattended while moderately "sick" persons receive treatment. This selection is clearly based on social criteria, not on psychiatric ones.

The layman usually assumes that his conception of "mental illness" is not the important definition, since the psychiatrist is the expert and presumably makes the final decision. On the contrary, community persons are brought to the hospital on the basis of lay definitions, and once they arrive, their appearance alone is usually regarded as sufficient evidence of "illness."

In the crowded state or county hospitals, which is the most typical situation, the psychiatrist does not have sufficient time to make a very complete psychiatric diagnosis, nor do his psychiatric tools provide him with the equipment for an expeditious screening of the patient. If he is a psychiatrist trained in the more orthodox psychoanalytic notions, his belief system makes it impossible to determine the "sickness" or "wellness" of the patient, since the classical theories assume that all people have unconscious drives which interfere with optimal functioning, and no clear practical criteria are provided for judging the "sick" from the "well."

In the two mental hospitals studied over a period of three months, the investigator never observed a case where the psychiatrist advised the patient that he did not need treatment. Rather, all persons who appeared at the hospital were absorbed into the patient population regardless of their ability to function adequately outside the hospital.

In this regard, it is important to note that mental hospitals care for more than the mentally ill. The unwanted, the aged, the indigent, the lonely, and others often enter public mental hospitals voluntarily. For example, on an alcoholic ward in a hospital studied by the author, staff generally recognized that as weather became cold and as snow began falling, indigent alcoholics would enter the hospital voluntarily, only to return to their usual patterns of life when the weather improved.

Psychiatric hospitals filled well over capacity will attempt to control more carefully those they will accept for treatment. But should beds be available, as was the case with the hospitals studied, it is likely that they will absorb whoever appears, at least for a time. This suggests that the definition of "mental illness" made by the lay public is crucial with regard to who is treated, and comprehension of medical care programs requires an understanding of how such definitions are made.

Intervention in a situation of "assumed mental illness" by family, friends, and others in the community is highly dependent on the visibility of symptoms.[5] Persons recognized and treated may not be those most in need of treatment by psychiatric criteria. Rather, it is at the point at which deviancy is most easily and clearly recognized—and most disturbing to the group—that pressures of various sorts are brought to bear on the person. Intervention, then, is likely to occur only after the person becomes a problem to himself or others, or gives definite indications that he will soon be a problem.

In evaluating the criteria by which visible symptoms might be judged, one practical basis is the extent to which the person failed to fulfill expectations adequately in performing his primary social roles (especially his familial and occupational roles), and the extent to which he violated legal and moral norms and highly important values of the group.

Whether a definition of deviancy is made and acted upon will depend largely on how serious the consequences of this deviation are for the group.[6] Some deviant behaviors are rewarded and tolerated. Others have some idiosyncratic function for the group, as is often the case with the "comic." Perhaps the deviant may be thought of as "eccentric," "queer," or "strange" but not sufficiently so to merit a definition of illness. However, should the deviancy begin to have serious consequences, because it is damaging or harmful to the individual, a group, or both, or because it becomes so visible to external groups that the family suffers loss of status, it might be redefined as "mental illness" and the person sent for treatment.

In some groups, of course, the stigma attached to a definition of mental illness is sufficiently great to bring about group resistance to such a definition.[7] However, other factors being constant, a definition of "mental illness" is more likely to be made as the serious consequences of the deviancy increase.[8]

The size and form of social structure characteristic of a community can affect the visibility of symptomatology, hence its consequences and definition. The data relevant to this area, however, are not very clear. It appears that in the autonomy of a large and impersonal network of relationships, the social visibility of persons lessens and symptoms may not be defined as readily as in more intimate communities. However, in the latter case, where the demands of social life may not be as rigorous and the deviant may not be as much of an inconvenience, the behavior is more likely to be ignored or tolerated, and the deviant can perform useful social roles more readily. In the larger and more impersonal structures, the abilities required to obtain sufficient life gratifications may be greater, and the person handicapped in his interpersonal responses may have a more difficult time making a satisfactory adjustment to life demands.[9]

The visibility and consequences of deviancy also increase as the deviant act increases in frequency. Other factors being equal, the frequency of a deviant act will affect how likely it is to be noticed, defined, and acted upon. Moreover, as the deviant act increases in frequency, it becomes more annoying to the group and some sanction is more likely to follow.

Depending upon life circumstances, groups—both family and community—differ in the kinds and degree of toleration they have for various behaviors. When the vulnerability of the group increases, its toleration for deviancy decreases.[10] During stress situations and crises, vulnerability increases, group solidarity becomes more essential, and deviation is treated more harshly, especially where the deviation exacerbates the crisis and further increases group vulnerability.

Moreover, during periods of family and community stress,

deviancy may increase because already handicapped persons find themselves unable to cope with the new and rigorous demands made upon them.

There are occasions when a person's behaviors, while tolerated in the primary group, become visible to authorities in the persons secondary groups who may have different values and standards. Hence there are different toleration levels for various behaviors, and those who define these behaviors as signs of "mental illness" may forcefully bring the patient to a treatment center.[11]

When this occurs, the primary group sometimes resists the definition placed upon its member by the secondary authorities; and it is not unusual for conflicting definitions to arise among the patient, his family, the courts, and the hospital physician. While the court is likely to accept the professional opinion of the physician, there are occasions when the psychiatrist—who by independent criteria has either assumed or decided that serious pathology exists—insists that a patient is ill, while the patient and his family strongly resist this definition. In such cases, the physician is often reluctant to press his definition and urge court commitment, since this requires him to argue in some states that the patient is dangerous to himself and others, a contention which is very difficult to support in many cases. In these state institutions, when the physician does decide to press such a petition for the commitment of an unwilling patient, his decision is usually made on the basis of whether there is sufficient evidence to convince the court that the patient should be lawfully detained, even when the family is reluctant.

Often the patient is released from the hospital without detailed judicial consideration, not because the psychiatrist finds him free of serious pathology, but rather because the psychiatrist has anticipated what the court decision would be. If the psychiatrist is to gain commitment of an unwilling patient, he must usually convince the family that the patient is indeed seriously ill and in need of treatment, and bring them around to support his definition of the situation.

In any case, the psychiatrist treating a patient implicitly, if not explicitly, recognizes that it is important to communicate his perception of pathology to the patient and to his family.

He also realizes that he must convince the patient that he is indeed "sick" and in serious need of treatment. The necessity of having the patient accept the psychiatric definition of his case is especially apparent in the early hospital experience, where the patient must become socialized to a "patient-role," accepting the definition of his symptoms placed upon him by the hospital population, including staff and other patients. Should the patient refuse to accept the patient-role and deny his illness, this resistance is viewed as a further symptom of the "illness," and he is told that if he is to get well, he must recognize the fact that he is ill.

Should the patient continue to reject the psychiatric definition of his illness, the psychiatrist is likely to report that the patient is a poor treatment risk. Furthermore, ancillary hospital staff and other patients also apply similar definitions of illness to the patient and expect him to accept these definitions. The patient's denials create social difficulties for him within the hospital, difficulties of adaptation to ward life which can be further viewed as indications that the patient is seriously ill and which reinforce the original impressions and definitions placed upon him by physicians, aides and other patients. Unless the patient begins to see himself through the eyes of the psychiatrist, hospital personnel, and other patients, he will remain a problem to the ward, and his therapy and progress are likely to be viewed as inconsequential.[12]

The foregoing suggests that if we are to understand the "mentally ill" patient, we must understand the situation from which he comes and the circumstances that led to the definition that he needs treatment. If the patient is to be effectively treated in regard to his life situation, we must understand what demands were made upon him and why he failed to meet these demands. Was it because he was unable to perceive the expectations of others accurately? Was it because he was unable to make proper responses? Or were there other reasons for his failure to meet expectations? Furthermore, we should want to inquire about the expectations he faced, the conflicts he perceived, and the cross-currents of expectations and behaviors that led to the societal response and definitions of mental illness.

From a theoretical point of view, what has been attempted is a descriptive model of the definitional processes by which persons within a community are adjudged as mentally ill. If we are to expand our understanding of definitions of deviancy and mental illness, a logical step is to move in the direction of axiomatic models, utilizing relevant variables and encouraging systematic empirical investigation. It is with the constant interplay of exploratory observations, systematic theory, and rigorous empirical tests that our knowledge will develop in a useful fashion.*

The Psychological Meaning
of Mental Illness in the Family

*MARIAN RADKE YARROW, CHARLOTTE GREEN
SCHWARTZ, HARRIET S. MURPHY, AND
LEILA CALHOUN DEASY*

The manifestations of mental illness are almost as varied as the spectrum of human behavior. Moreover, they are expressed not only in disturbance and functional impairment for the sick person but also in disruptive interactions with others. The mentally ill person is often, in his illness, a markedly deviant person, though certainly less so than the popular stereotype of the "insane." One wonders what were the initial phases of the impact of mental illness upon those within the ill person's social environment. How were the

* The author wishes to express his thanks to Edmund Volkart and Thomas Scheff for their helpful comments.

FROM *The Journal of Social Issues*, XI, no. 4:12–24; 1955. Reprinted by permission of the authors and *The Journal of Social Issues*.

disorders of illness interpreted and tolerated? What did the patients, prior to hospitalization, communicate of their needs, and how did others—those closest to the ill persons—attempt, psychologically and behaviorally, to cope with the behavior? How did these persons come to be recognized by other family members as needing psychiatric help?

This paper presents an analysis of cognitive and emotional problems encountered by the wife in coping with the mental illness of the husband. It is concerned with the factors which lead to the reorganization of the wife's perceptions of her husband from a *well* man to a man who is mentally sick or in need of hospitalization in a mental hospital. The process whereby the wife attempts to understand and interpret her husband's manifestations of mental illness is best communicated by considering first the concrete details of a single wife's experiences. The findings and interpretations based on the total sample are presented following the case analysis.

ILLUSTRATIVE CASE

Robert F., a 35-year-old cab driver, was admitted to Saint Elizabeth's Hospital with a diagnosis of schizophrenia. How did Mr. F. get to the mental hospital? Here is a very condensed version of what his wife told an interviewer a few weeks later.

Mrs. F. related certain events, swift and dramatic, which led directly to the hospitalization. The day before admission, Mr. F. went shopping with his wife, which he never had done before, and expressed worry lest he lose her. This was in her words, "rather strange." (*His behavior is not in keeping with her expectations for him.*) Later that day, Mr. F. thought a TV program was about him and that the set was "after him." "Then I was getting worried." (*She recognizes the bizarre nature of his reactions. She becomes concerned.*)

That night, Mr. F. kept talking. He reproached himself for not working enough to give his wife surprises. Suddenly, he exclaimed he did have a surprise for her—he was going to kill her. "I was petrified and said to him, 'What do you mean?' Then, he began to cry and told me not to let him hurt me and to do for him what I would want him to do for me. I asked him what was wrong. He said he had cancer. . . . He began talking about his grandfather's mustache and said there was a worm growing out of it." She remembered his watching little worms in the fish bowl and thought his idea came from that. Mr. F. said he had killed his grandfather. He asked Mrs. F. to forgive him and wondered if she were his mother or God. She denied this. He vowed he was being punished for killing people during the war. "I thought maybe... worrying about the war so much... had gotten the best of him. (*She tries to understand his behavior. She stretches the range of normality to include it.*) I thought he should see a psychiatrist... I don't know how to explain it. He was shaking. I knew it was beyond what I could do... I was afraid of him... I thought he was losing his normal mental attitude and mentality, but I wouldn't say that he was insane or crazy, because he had always bossed me around before...." (*She shifts back and forth in thinking his problem is psychiatric and in feeling it is normal behavior that could be accounted for in terms of their own experience.*) Mr. F. talked on through the night. Sometime in the morning, he "seemed to straighten out" and drove his wife to work. (*This behavior tends to balance out the preceding disturbed activities. She quickly returns to a normal referent.*)

At noon, Mr. F. walked into the store where his wife worked as a clerk. "I couldn't make any sense of what he was saying. He kept getting angry because I wouldn't talk to him.... Finally, the boss' wife told me to go home." En route, Mr. F. said his male organs were blown up and little seeds covered him. Mrs. F. denied seeing them and announced she planned to call his mother. "He began crying and I had to promise not to. I said,... 'Don't you think you should go to a psychiatrist?' and he said, 'No, there is nothing wrong with me.'... Then we came home, and I went to pay a bill...." (*Again she considers, but is not fully committed to, the idea that psychiatric help is needed.*)

Back at their apartment, Mr. F. talked of repairing his cab while Mrs. F. thought of returning to work and getting someone to call a doctor. Suddenly, he started chasing her around the apartment and growling like a lion. Mrs. F. screamed, Mr. F. ran out of the apartment, and Mrs. F. slammed and locked the door. "When he started roaring and growling, then I thought he was crazy. That wasn't a human sound. You couldn't say a thing to him...." Later, Mrs. F. learned that her husband went to a nearby church, created a scene, and was taken to the hospital by the police. (*Thoroughly threatened, she defines problem as psychiatric.*)

What occurred before these events which precipitated the hospitalization? Going back to their early married life, approximately three years before hospitalization, Mrs. F. told of her husband's irregular work habits and long-standing complaints of severe headaches. "When we were first married, he didn't work much and I didn't worry as long as we could pay the bills." Mrs. F. figured they were just married and wanted to be together a lot. (*Personal norms and expectations are built up.*)

At Thanksgiving, six months after marriage, Mr. F. "got sick and stopped working." During the war he contracted malaria, he explained, which always recurred at that time of year. "He wouldn't get out of bed or eat.... He thought he was constipated and he had nightmares.... What I noticed most was his perspiring so much. He was crabby. You couldn't get him to go to a doctor. . . . I noticed he was nervous. He's always been a nervous person. . . . Any little thing that would go wrong would upset him—if I didn't get a drawer closed right. . . . His friends are nervous, too. . . . I came to the conclusion that maybe I was happy-go-lucky and everyone else was a bundle of nerves. . . . For a cab driver, he worked hard—most cab drivers loaf. When he felt good, he worked hard. He didn't work so hard when he didn't." (*She adapts to his behavior. The atypical is normalized as his type of personality and appropriate to his subculture.*)

As the months and years went by, Mrs. F. changed jobs frequently, but she worked more regularly than did her husband. He continued to work sporadically, get sick intermittently, appear "nervous and tense" and refrain from seeking medical care. Mrs. F. "couldn't say what was wrong." She had first one idea, then another, about his behavior. "I knew it wasn't right for him to be acting sick like he did." Then, "I was beginning to think he was getting lazy because there wasn't anything I could see." During one period, Mrs. F. surmised he was carrying on with another woman. "I was right on the verge of going, until he explained it wasn't anyone else." (*There is a building up of deviant behavior to a point near her tolerance limits. Her interpretations shift repeatedly.*)

About two and a half years before admission, Mrs. F. began talking to friends about her husband's actions and her lack of success in getting him to a doctor. "I got disgusted and said if he didn't go to a doctor, I would leave him. I got Bill (the owner of Mr. F.'s cab) to talk to him. . . . I begged, threatened, fussed. . . ." After that, Mr. F. went to a VA doctor for one visit, overslept for his second appointment and never returned. He said the doctor told him nothing was wrong.

When Mr. F. was well and working, Mrs. F. "never stopped to think about it." "You live from day to day. . . . When something isn't nice, I don't think about it. If you stop to think about things, you can worry yourself sick. . . . He said he wished he could live in my world. He'd never seem to be able to put his thinking off the way I do. . . ." (*Her mode of operating permits her to tolerate his behavior.*)

Concurrently, other situations confronted Mrs. F. Off and on, Mr. F. talked of a coming revolution as a result of which Negroes and Jews would take over the world. If Mrs. F. argued that she didn't believe it, Mr. F. called her "dumb" and "stupid." "The best thing to do was to change the subject." Eighteen months before admission, Mr. F. began awakening his wife to tell of nightmares about wartime experiences, but she "didn't think about it." Three months later, he decided he wanted to do something besides drive a cab. He worked on an invention but discovered it was patented. Then, he began to write a book about his wartime experiences and science. "If you saw what he wrote, you couldn't see anything wrong with it. . . . He just wasn't making any money." Mrs. F. did think it was "silly" when Mr. F. went to talk to Einstein about his ideas and couldn't understand why he didn't talk to someone in town. Nevertheless, she accompanied him on the trip. (*With the further accumulation of deviant behavior, she becomes less*

*and less able to tolerate it. The perceived seriousness of his condition is
attenuated so long as she is able to find something acceptable or understandable in his behavior.*)

Three days before admission, Mr. F. stopped taking baths and changing clothes. Two nights before admission, he awakened his wife to tell
her he had just figured out that the book he was writing had nothing
to do with science or the world, only with himself. "He said he had
been worrying about things for ten years and that writing a book
solved what had been worrying him for ten years." Mrs. F. told him to
burn his writings if they had nothing to do with science. It was the
following morning that Mrs. F. first noticed her husband's behavior as
"rather strange."

In the long prelude to Mr. F.'s hospitalization, one can see
many of the difficulties which arise for the wife as the
husband's behavior no longer conforms and as it strains the
limits of the wife's expectations for him. At some stage the
wife defines the situation as one requiring help, eventually
psychiatric help. Our analysis is concerned primarily with
the process of the wife's getting to this stage in interpreting
and responding to the husband's behavior. In the preceding
case are many reactions which appear as general trends in
the data group. These trends can be systematized in terms of
the following focal aspects of the process:

1. The wife's threshold for initially discerning a problem
depends on the accumulation of various kinds of behavior
which are not readily understandable or acceptable to her.

2. This accumulation forces upon the wife the necessity
for examining and adjusting expectations for herself and
her husband which permit her to account for his behavior.

3. The wife is in an "overlapping" situation, of problem
—not problem or of normal—not normal. Her interpretations
shift back and forth.

4. Adaptations to the atypical behavior of the husband
occur. There is testing and waiting for additional cues in
coming to any given interpretation, as in most problem
solving. The wife mobilizes strong defenses against the husband's deviant behavior. These defenses take form in such
reactions as denying, attenuating, balancing and normalizing
the husband's problems.

5. Eventually there is a threshold point at which the perception breaks, when the wife comes to the relatively stable

conclusion that the problem is a psychiatric one and/or that she cannot alone cope with the husband's behavior.

These processes are elaborated in the following analysis of the wives' responses.

METHOD OF DATA COLLECTION

Ideally, to study this problem one might like to interview the wives as they struggled with the developing illness. This is precluded, however, by the fact that the problem is not "visible" until psychiatric help is sought. The data, therefore, are the wives' reconstructions of their earlier experiences and accounts of their current reactions during the husband's hospitalization.

It is recognized that recollections of the prehospital period may well include systematic biases, such as distortions, omissions, and increased organization and clarity. As a reliability check, a number of wives, just before the husband's discharge from the hospital, were asked again to describe the events and feelings of the prehospital period. In general, the two reports are markedly similar; often details are added and others are elaborated, but events tend to be substantially the same. While this check attests to the consistency of the wives' reporting, it has, of course, the contamination of overlearning which comes from many retellings of these events.

THE BEGINNINGS OF THE WIFE'S CONCERN

In the early interviews, the wife was asked to describe the beginnings of the problem which led to her husband's hospitalization. ("Could you tell me when you first noticed that your husband was different?") This question was intended to provide an orientation for the wife to reconstruct the sequence and details of events and feelings which characterized the period preceding hospitalization. The interviewer provided a minimum of structuring in order that the wife's emphases and organization could be obtained.

In retrospect, the wives usually cannot pinpoint the time the husband's problem emerged. Neither can they clearly carve it out from the contexts of the husband's personality and family expectations. The subjective beginnings are seldom localized in a single strange or disturbing reaction on the husband's part but rather in the piling up of behavior and feelings. We have seen this process for Mrs. F. There is a similar accumulation for the majority of wives, although the time periods and kinds of reported behavior vary. Thus, Mrs. Q., verbalizes the impact of a concentration of changes which occur within a period of a few weeks. Her explicit recognition of a problem comes when she adds up this array: her husband stays out late, doesn't eat or sleep, has obscene thoughts, argues with her, hits her, talks continuously, "cannot appreciate the beautiful scene," and "cannot appreciate me or the baby."

The problem behaviors reported by the wives are given in Table 1. They are ordered roughly; the behaviors listed first occurred primarily, but not exclusively, within the family; those later occurred in the more public domain. Whether the behavior is public or private does not seem to be a very significant factor in determining the wife's threshold for perceiving a problem.

There are many indications that these behaviors, now organized as a problem, have occurred many times before. This is especially true where alcoholism, physical complaints, or personality "weaknesses" enter the picture. The wives indicate how, earlier, they had assimilated these characteristics into their own expectations in a variety of ways: the characteristics were congruent with their image of their husbands, they fitted their differential standards for men and women (men being less able to stand up to troubles), they had social or environmental justifications, etc.

When and how behavior becomes defined as problematic appears to be a highly individual matter. In some instances, it is when the wife can no longer manage her husband (he will no longer respond to her usual prods); in others, when his behavior destroys the status quo (when her goals and living routines are disorganized); and, in still others, when she cannot explain his behavior. One can speculate that her

TABLE 1. Reported Problem Behavior at Time of the Wife's Initial Concern and at Time of the Husband's Admission to Hospital

Problem Behavior	Initially		At Hospital Admission	
	Psychotics N	Psycho-neurotics N	Psychotics N	Psycho-neurotics N
Physical problems, complaints, worries	12	5	7	5
Deviations from routines of behavior	17	9	13	9
Expressions of inadequacy or hopelessness	4	1	5	2
Nervous, irritable, worried	19	10	18	9
Withdrawal (verbal, physical)	5	1	6	1
Changes or accentuations in personality "traits" (slovenly, deceptive, forgetful)	5	6	7	6
Aggressive or assaultive and suicidal behavior	6	3	10	6
Strange or bizarre thoughts, delusions, hallucinations and strange behavior	11	1	15	2
Excessive drinking	4	7	3	4
Violation of codes of "decency"	3	1	3	2
NUMBER OF RESPONDENTS	23	10	23	10

level of tolerance for his behavior is a function of her specific personality needs and vulnerabilities, her personal and family value system, and the social supports and prohibitions regarding the husband's symptomatic behavior.

INITIAL INTERPRETATIONS OF HUSBAND'S PROBLEM

Once the behavior is organized as a problem, it tends also to be interpreted as some particular kind of problem. More often than not, however, the husband's difficulties are not seen initially as manifestations of mental illness or even as emotional problems (Table 2).

TABLE 2.   Initial Interpretations of the Husband's Behavior

Interpretation	Psychotics N	Psychoneurotics N
Nothing really wrong	3	0
"Character" weakness and "controllable" behavior (lazy, mean, etc.)	6	3
Physical problem	6	0
Normal response to crisis	3	1
Mildly emotionally disturbed	1	2
"Something" seriously wrong	2	2
Serious emotional or mental problem	2	2
NUMBER OF RESPONDENTS	23	10

Early interpretations often tend to be organized around physical difficulties (18 percent of cases) or "character" problems (27 percent). To a very marked degree, these orientations grow out of the wives' long-standing appraisals of their husbands as weak and ineffective or physically sick men. These wives describe their husbands as spoiled, lacking will power, exaggerating little complaints, and acting like babies. This is especially marked where alcoholism complicates the husband's symptomatology. For example, Mrs. Y., whose husband was chronically alcoholic, aggressive and threatening to her, "raving," and who "chewed his nails until they almost bled," interprets his difficulty thus: "He was just spoiled rotten. He never outgrew it. He told me when he was a child he could get his own way if he insisted, and he is still that way." This quotation is the prototype of many of its kind.

Some wives, on the other hand, locate the problem in the environment. They expect the husband to change as the environmental crisis subsides. Several wives, while enumerating difficulties and concluding that there is a problem, in the same breath say it is really nothing to be concerned about.

Where the wives interpret the husband's difficulty as emotional in nature, they tend to be inconsistently "judgmental" and "understanding." The psychoneurotics are more often perceived initially by their wives as having emotional problems or as being mentally ill than are the psychotics. This is true even though many more clinical signs (bizarre, confused, delusional, aggressive, and disoriented behavior) are reported by the wives of the psychotics than of the psychoneurotics.

Initial interpretations, whatever their content, are seldom held with great confidence by the wives. Many recall their early reactions to their husbands' behaviors as full of puzzling confusion and uncertainty. Something is wrong, they know, but, in general, they stop short of a firm explanation. Thus, Mrs. M. reports, "He was kind of worried. He was kind of worried before, not exactly worried. . . ." She thought of his many physical complaints; she "racked" her "brain" and told her husband, "Of course, he didn't feel good." Finally, he stayed home from work with "no special complaints, just blah," and she "began to realize it was more deeply seated."

CHANGING PERCEPTIONS OF THE HUSBAND'S PROBLEM

The fog and uneasiness in the wife's early attempts to understand and cope with the husband's difficulties are followed, typically, by painful psychological struggles to resolve the uncertainties and to change the current situation. Usually, the wife's perceptions of the husband's problems undergo a series of changes before hospitalization is sought or effected, irrespective of the length of time elapsing between the beginnings of concern and hospitalization.

Viewing these changes macroscopically, three relatively distinct patterns of successive redefinitions of the husband's problems are apparent. One sequence (slightly less than half the cases) is characterized by a progressive intensification; interpretations are altered in a definite direction—toward seeing the problem as mental illness. Mrs. O. illustrates this progression. Initially, she thought her husband was "unsure of himself." "He was worried, too, about getting old." These ideas moved to: "He'd drink to forget. . . . He just didn't have

the confidence. . . . He'd forget little things. . . . He'd wear a
suit weeks on end if I didn't take it away from him. . . . He'd
say nasty things." Then, when Mr. O. seemed "so confused,"
"to forget all kinds of things . . . where he'd come from . . .
to go to work," and made "nasty, cutting remarks all the
time," she began to think in terms of a serious personality
disturbance. "I did think he knew that something was
wrong . . . that he was sick. He was never any different this
last while and I couldn't stand it any more. . . . You don't
know what a relief it was . . . " (when he was hospitalized).
The husband's drinking, his failure to be tidy, his nastiness,
etc., lose significance in their own right. They move from
emphasis to relief and are recast as signs of "something
deeper," something that brought "it" on.

Some wives whose interpretations move in the direction of
seeing their husbands as mentally ill hold conceptions of
mental illness and of personality that do not permit assigning
the husband all aspects of the sick role. Frequently, they use
the interpretation of mental illness as an angry epithet or
as a threatening prediction for the husband. This is exemplified in such references as: "I told him he should have his
head examined," "I called him a half-wit," "I told him if he's
not careful, he'll be a mental case." To many of these wives,
the hospital is regarded as the "end of the road."

Other wives showing this pattern of change hold conceptions of emotional disturbance which more easily permit
them to assign to their husbands the role of patient as the
signs of illness become more apparent. They do not so often
regard hospitalization in a mental hospital as the "last step."
Nevertheless, their feelings toward their husbands may contain components equally as angry and rejecting as those of
the wives with the less sophisticated ideas regarding mental
illness.

A somewhat different pattern of sequential changes in
interpreting the husband's difficulties (about one-fifth of the
cases) is to be found among wives who appear to cast around
for situationally and momentarily adequate explanations. As
the situation changes or as the husband's behavior changes,
these wives find reasons and excuses but lack an underlying

or synthesizing theory. Successive interpretations tend to bear little relation to one another. Situational factors tend to lead them to seeing their husbands as mentally ill. Immediate, serious, and direct physical threats or the influence of others may be the deciding factor. For example, a friend or employer may insist that the husband see a psychiatrist, and the wife goes along with the decision.

A third pattern of successive redefinitions (slightly less than one-third of the cases) revolves around an orientation outside the framework of emotional problems or mental illness. In these cases, the wife's specific explanations change but pivot around a denial that the husband is mentally ill.

A few wives seem not to change their interpretations about their husband's difficulties. They maintain the same explanation throughout the development of his illness, some within the psychiatric framework, others rigidly outside that framework.

Despite the characteristic shiftings in interpretations, in the group as a whole, there tend to be persisting underlying themes in the individual wife's perceptions that remain essentially unaltered. These themes are a function of her systems of thinking about normality and abnormality and about valued and devalued behavior.

THE PROCESS OF RECOGNIZING THE HUSBAND'S PROBLEM AS MENTAL ILLNESS

In the total situation confronting the wife, there are a number of factors, apparent in our data, which make it difficult for the wife to recognize and accept the husband's behavior in a mental-emotional-psychiatric framework. Many crosscurrents seem to influence the process.

The husband's behavior itself is a fluctuating stimulus. He is not worried and complaining all of the time. His delusions and hallucinations may not persist. His hostility toward the wife may be followed by warm attentiveness. She has, then, the problem of deciding whether his "strange" behavior is significant. The greater saliency of one or the other of his responses at any moment of time depends in some degree upon the behavior sequence which has occurred most recently.

The relationship between husband and wife also supplies a variety of images and contexts which can justify varied conclusions about the husband's current behavior. The wife is likely to adapt to behavior which occurs in their day to day relationships. Therefore, symptomatic reactions which are intensifications of long-standing response patterns become part of the fabric of life and are not easily disentangled as "symptomatic."

Communications between husband and wife regarding the husband's difficulties act sometimes to impede and sometimes to further the process of seeing the difficulties within a psychiatric framework. We have seen both kinds of influences in our data. Mr. and Mrs. F. were quite unable to communicate effectively about Mr. F.'s problems. On the one hand, he counters his wife's urging that he see a doctor with denials that anything is wrong. On the other hand, in his own way through his symptoms, he tries to communicate his problems, but she responds only to his verbalized statements, taking them at face value.

Mr. and Mrs. K. participate together quite differently, examining Mr. K.'s fears that he is being followed by the F.B.I., that their house has been wired, and that he is going to be fired. His wife tentatively shares his suspicions. At the same time, they discuss the possibility of paranoid reactions.

The larger social context contributes, too, in the wife's perceptual tug of war. Others with whom she can compare her husband provide contrasts to his deviance, but others (Mr. F.'s nervous friends) also provide parallels to his problems. The "outsiders," seeing less of her husband, often discount the wife's alarm when she presses them for opinions. In other instances, the friend or employer, less adapted to or defended against the husband's symptoms, helps her to define his problem as psychiatric.

This task before the wife, of defining her husband's difficulties, can be conceptualized as an "overlapping" situation (in Lewin's terms), in which the relative potencies of the several effective influences fluctuate. The wife is responding to the various sets of forces simultaneously. Thus, several conclusions or interpretations of the problem are simultaneously "suspended in balance," and they shift back and forth in emphasis and relief. Seldom, however, does she seem to be balancing off clear-cut alternatives, such as physical versus mental. Her complex perceptions (even those of Mrs. F., who is extreme in misperceiving cues) are more "sophisticated" than the casual questioner might be led to conclude.

Thus far, we have ignored the personally threatening aspects of recognizing mental illness in one's spouse, and the defenses which are mobilized to meet this threat. It is assumed that it is threatening to the wife not only to realize that the husband is mentally ill but further to consider her own possible role in the development of the disorder, to give up modes of relating to her husband that may have had satisfactions for her and to see a future as the wife of a mental patient. Our data provide systematic information only on the first aspect of this problem, on the forms of defense against the recognition of the illness. One or more of the following defenses are manifested in three-fourths of our cases.

The most obvious form of defense in the wife's response is the tendency to *normalize* the husband's neurotic and psychotic symptoms. His behavior is explained, justified or made acceptable by seeing it also in herself or by assuring herself that the particular behavior occurs again and again among persons who are not ill. Illustrative of this reaction is the wife who reports her husband's hallucinations and assures herself that this is normal because she herself heard voices when she was in the menopause. Another wife responds to her husband's physical complaints, fears, worries, nightmares and delusions with "A lot of normal people think there's something wrong when there isn't. I think men are that way; his father is that way."

When behavior cannot be normalized, it can be made to seem less severe or less important in a total picture than an outsider might see it. By finding some grounds for the behavior or something explainable about it, the wife achieves at least momentary *attenuation* of the seriousness of it. Thus, Mrs. F. is able to discount partly the strangeness of her husband's descriptions of the worms growing out of his grandfather's mustache when she recalls his watching the worms in the fish bowl. There may be attenuation, too, by seeing the behavior as "momentary" ("You could talk him out of his ideas") or by rethinking the problem and seeing it in a different light.

By *balancing* acceptable with unacceptable behavior or "strange" with "normal" behavior, some wives can conclude that the husband is not seriously disturbed. Thus, it is very important to Mrs. R. that her husband kissed her goodbye before he left for the hospital. This response cancels out his hostile feelings toward her and the possibility that he is mentally ill. Similarly, Mrs. V. reasons that her husband cannot be "out of his mind" for he had reminded her of things she must not forget to do when he went to the hospital.

Defense sometimes amounts to a thorough-going *denial*. This takes the form of denying that the behavior perceived can be interpreted in an emotional or psychiatric framework. In some instances, the wife reports vividly on such behavior as repeated thoughts of suicide, efforts to harm her and the like and sums it up with "I thought it was just a whim." Other wives bend their efforts toward proving the implausibility of mental illness.

After the husband is hospitalized, it might be expected that these denials would decrease to a negligible level. This is not wholly the case, however. A breakdown of the wives' interpretations just following the husband's admission to the hospital shows that roughly a fifth still interpret the husband's behavior in another framework than that of a serious emotional problem or mental illness. Another fifth ambivalently and sporadically interpret the behavior as an emotional or mental problem. The remainder hold relatively stable interpretations within this framework.

After the husband has been hospitalized for some time, many wives reflect on their earlier tendencies to avoid a definition of mental illness. Such reactions are almost identically described by these wives: "I put it out of my mind— I didn't want to face it—anything but a mental illness." "Maybe I was aware of it. But you know you push things away from you and keep hoping." "Now you think maybe you should have known about it. Maybe you should have done more than you did and that worries me."

DISCUSSION

The findings on the perceptions of mental illness by the wives of patients are in line with general findings in studies of perception. Behavior which is unfamiliar and incongruent and unlikely in terms of current expectations and needs will not be readily recognized, and stressful or threatening stimuli will tend to be misperceived or perceived with difficulty or delay.

We have attempted to describe the factors which help the wife maintain a picture of her husband as normal and those which push her in the direction of accepting a psychiatric definition of his problem. The kind and intensity of the symptomatic behavior, its persistence over time, the husband's interpretation of his problem, interpretations and defining actions of others, including professionals, all play a role. In addition, the wives come to this experience with different conceptions of psychological processes and of the nature of emotional illness, itself, as well as with different tolerances for emotional disturbance. As we have seen, there are also many supports in society for maintaining a picture of normality concerning the husband's behavior. Social pressures and expectations not only keep *behavior* in line but to a great extent *perceptions* of behavior as well.

There are implications of these findings both for those who are working in the field of prevention of mental illness and early detection of emotional disturbance as well as for the rehabilitation worker. They suggest that to acquaint the public with the nature of mental illness by describing psychotic behavior and emphasizing its nonthreatening aspect is, after all, an intellectualization and not likely to be effective in dealing with the threatening aspects of recognizing mental illness which we have described. Further, it is not enough simply to recognize the fact that the rehabilitation of patients is affected by the attitudes and feelings of the family toward the patient and his illness. Perhaps a better acceptance of the patient can be developed if families who have been unable to deal with the problem of the illness are helped to work through this experience and to deal with their difficulties in accepting the illness and what remains of it after the patient leaves the hospital.

What the Mass Media Present

JUM C. NUNNALLY, JR.

The media of mass communication are commonly thought to exert a powerful influence on what the general public feels and believes. Consequently, we studied presentations dealing with mental-health phenomena in the mass media and the impact of the media on public opinion. This chapter will describe a content analysis of the mass media. . . .

CONTENT-ANALYSIS PROCEDURE

Content analysis is a counting operation. Examples of things that might be counted are the number of metaphors in Shakespearean plays, the number of friendly references to a political candidate in newspapers, and the number of times that a propaganda source refers to a particular issue. Our content analysis counted the number of times that particular points of view about mental health were portrayed in samples of mass-media presentations.[1]

From *Popular Conceptions of Mental Health*, Holt, Rinehart, and Winston, New York, 1961, 65–89. Reprinted by permission of the author and publisher.

Coding Categories

In a content analysis, the people who do the counting are referred to as *coders* and the things that they count are referred to as *coding categories*. Usually coding categories are determined a priori, or "rationally," rather than deduced from empirical observations. Our content analysis departed from the customary dependence on "rational" categories. One of the principles which guided our study of information held by our three sources (the public, the experts, and the media) was that comparable measures should be used for all three. Consequently, the ten information factors that were used to study the public and the experts were also used to study the content of the media.

How the information factors were used to analyze the content of media presentations can be illustrated with one of the television programs "caught" in our sample. The program was a 15-minute crime drama. As the scene opens, a thief is sneaking through a clock shop. The shop is filled with ticking clocks and swinging pendulums. The thief enters a barred enclave in the room where the "safe" is placed. The barred door accidently closes and locks, and the unfortunate thief must spend the night looking at and listening to a room full of clocks. When the proprietors arrive in the morning, the thief is staring glassy-eyed and mumbling incoherently. In the final scene he is carted away to a mental hospital.

How the content of this television presentation was analyzed will illustrate our general procedures. It was first necessary to decide whether any relevant material occurred. (How relevance was determined will be discussed later.) Relevant material was then "coded" on the ten information factors. A judgment was made as to whether the material affirmed each factor, repudiated each factor, or portrayed a neutral viewpoint (a neutral presentation either said or portrayed nothing relating to the ten factors or was a balance of pro and con). Scores of "plus," "minus," and "zero" were given for the results.

The television drama described above is relevant to our problem because the thief was referred to several times as being "out of his mind" and because he was placed in a mental hospital. The presentation was particularly relevant to two of our factors, "look and act different" (Factor I) and "immediate external environment versus personality dynamics" (Factor VII). The thief assumed a very bizarre appearance, which, if characteristic of the mentally ill at all, would be found only in the most severely ill. Consequently, the program was scored "plus" on Factor I. In the drama, the thief was "driven mad" by the ticking clocks. He entered the shop an apparently normal person (except for an unfortunate occupation) and left with a severe mental illness. The lesson that people might learn from this (fortunately people know better) is that one harrowing experience will bring on mental illness. Consequently, the program was scored "plus" on Factor VII. The details of the program supplied information enough to score some of the other information factors as either "plus" or "minus," and zeros were given to the remaining information factors because no related ideas were presented.

In addition to the ten factors, five supplementary content categories were employed. Counts were made of the number of portrayals of *supernatural* causes and cures associated with mental-health problems. Although supernatural explanations were generally rejected by the public, it was thought that some of the media presentations might deal with evil omens, visions, magic spells, and the like. The second supplementary category concerned the *approval of mental-health professions and facilities*. A "plus" was recorded if the portrayal suggested, for example, that psychiatrists usually do an effective job. An example of a "minus" situation is one in which the psychiatrist was in league with crooks and used his position to confine hapless victims in a mental hospital. Similarly, codings were made of portrayals relating to psychotherapy, mental hospitals, and specific forms of treatment. The third supplementary category concerned the *incidence* of mental-health problems: whether or not the presentation suggested that mental-health problems occur frequently in our society. For the fourth supplementary category, *methods of prevention and treatment*, coders simply listed all the suggested methods encountered in the media presentations. For the fifth supplementary category, *whom to approach for help* when mental problems occur, coders listed the kinds of persons suggested in the media presentations, such as ministers, psychiatrists, and lawyers.

In addition to the content categories, coders applied a number of space and time categories. For the printed media, the coders determined the amount of space taken up by each relevant message. For radio and television, coders noted the amount of time consumed by each relevant presentation— an hour, a half-hour, or only five minutes. The space and time categories were broken down in terms of the places in which relevant material appeared. For example, in the analysis of newspapers, each relevant item was classified into one of the following "location" categories: (1) news stories, features, and pictures, (2) paid advertising, (3) entertainment such as fiction, comics, and puzzles, (4) personal-advice columns on health and psychology and for the "lovelorn," (5) editorials, including political cartoons and "letters to the editor," and (6) all factual "how to" items, such as recipes, financial guides, and home-repair columns.

The ten factors and the supplementary categories were intended to measure the information stated and implied by mass-media presentations. In addition to these information-type measures, part of the content analysis was concerned with the attitudes suggested by the media presentations. For this, coders were asked to make judgments about the portrayals of the mentally ill and the persons who treated the mentally ill. Each character appearing in the media was rated on a series of seven-step attitude scales. The scales were bounded by polar adjectives such as safe-dangerous, strong-weak, and valuable-worthless. (This type of attitude-measuring instrument was used widely in our studies. . . .) The coders were not asked to rate their personal reactions to the characters portrayed but to try to make impartial judgments about the nature of the portrayals themselves.

Coder Selection and Training

The main job of the coders was to analyze media content on the basis of the ten information factors. Consequently, the coders had to be familiar with psychological concepts.

Six undergraduate majors in psychology were employed as coders, and a psychology graduate student supervised their work. The coders were given six hours of training. The meanings of the information factors were explained in detail, and the coders practiced using the factors. One form of practice was to make a "blind" sorting of the 180 information items (the ones used in the original factor analysis) into their proper factors. Thus, given a statement like "The eyes of the insane are glassy," the coders had to guess the corresponding factor (in this case the correct answer was Factor I, "look and act different"). On the average the coders assigned 75-percent of the items correctly, giving us some confidence in their understanding and use of the factors. As another form of practice, the coders made content analyses of excerpts from newspaper articles and of contrived written messages. The results were compared with the codings made by psychologists on the research staff, which resulted in more exact specification of the procedures of analysis and continued training for coders.

Media Samples

A truly representative sampling of the content of the mass media would be an enormous research undertaking. Not only are there numerous arms of the media (films, books, newspapers, radio, television, and others), but there are numerous classifications of each. Even a representative sample of one arm alone, such as magazines, would require a diverse and extensive collection. In comparison to a truly representative sampling of media content, our sample was relatively weak.

TELEVISION. Television coverage was the most restricted of our media samples, because of the difficulties and expenses of content-analyzing television programs as compared to newspapers, magazines, and other media. The television sample was restricted to the total output—about 111 hours of transmission time—of a single VHF station, WCIA in Champaign, Illinois, for one full week, January 31 through February 6, 1955. In addition to local productions, this station offered more than 100 CBS, nearly 20 NBC, and several DuMont programs.

As was true in all of the content analyses, every minute of the telecasting was considered for material relevant to mental health. Thus our coders watched such apparently unrelated presentations as basketball games, stock-market quotations, and commercials, but we did not want to judge in advance where relevant presentations would be found.

Coders worked in shifts to analyze television programs, with one shift of three coders watching at all times. A room equipped with clocks, two television sets (in case one fell into disrepair), and partitions separating the coders from one another was specially prepared for the analysis. Supervisors were available to distribute and collect coding sheets and to answer coders' questions about technical procedures.

RADIO. The radio sample consisted of one week's total broadcasting by four stations, affiliated with four different networks, in four widely separated geographic areas of the United States. The broadcasts had been recorded in November and December, 1953 for another project.[2] It proved much less tedious to analyze the radio recordings than it was to analyze "live" television. The coders were also able to play back portions of the program recordings to help them form judgments about the content categories.

MAGAZINES. In this sample were 91 different magazines, one issue of each, which were displayed on newsstands at about the same time in March, 1955. These included comic books, news, pictorial, digest, "quality," health, women's, men's, teen-age, sports, farm, romance and confession, detective, film, and other magazines. We tried to gather as diverse a collection as possible, excluding only such highly specialized magazines as photography and "how to" publications. About 351,000 column inches of space were included.

NEWSPAPERS. Our newspaper sample was both the most extensive and the most representative for the country as a whole. The sample consisted of one week's "home" editions of 49 daily newspapers. The newspapers were proportionately representative of the geographic regions in the United States and proportionately representative of circulation size. The issues were spread over the month of October, 1954. Involved were 317 separate issues with a total of 12,419 pages, containing approximately 2,086,423 inches—and every inch was searched for material relating to mental health.

CONFESSION MAGAZINES. In gathering the magazine sample discussed above, we found that "confession" magazines are saturated with material relating to mental illness, neurosis, and emotional disturbance. Consequently, a separate study was made of the mental-health content of confession magazines.[3] Different methods of content analysis were used on the confession magazines and the results were not combined directly with those from our four other media samples.

Some Technical Details

The general logic for sampling the media and analyzing the content was relatively clear. As is usually the case, however, we had to solve some knotty practical problems in the actual research. Some of these technical details will be discussed in this section.

THE SCORING UNIT.   Before applying the content measures (the information factors, the supplementary categories, and the attitude ratings), we had to designate what the item, or the unit, for scoring would be. As a practical solution we defined units as separable programs in radio and television and separable "columns" in newspapers and magazines. Thus in radio or television, a half-hour comedy program, including commercials and other announcements, was scored as a whole and constituted a single item or unit. In magazines, a complete story or feature was considered a single item, including the continuation of the feature or story from page to page. If the story continued to another issue or if the feature reappeared regularly, the material in one issue was considered a single item, and the material occurring in subsequent issues was considered a new item. As for magazines, the entire content of each separable newspaper story and feature was considered as one unit. Some of the items or units in particular issues were an editorial column about the cold war, a syndicated short story, a Joe Palooka comic strip, an advertisement for television sets, and a front-page story about an airplane accident.

RELEVANCE OF CONTENT. The analysis consisted of a twofold set of decisions: first whether a particular excerpt from the media (a television program or a magazine story) contained material related to mental health, and, if so, how the material conformed to our coding categories (the information factors, the supplementary information categories, and the attitude ratings).

Relevance was determined on the basis of the definition of our project area: information and attitudes about mental disorder—the psychoses, the neuroses, and lesser disturbances. In choosing topics to study and in selecting relevant material from the media, we preferred to err toward over-inclusion rather than toward underinclusion. Consequently, our studies include some findings relating to child-rearing practices, alcoholism, juvenile delinquency, and other phenomena that are usually considered parts of mental health. We considered such matters as relevant, however, only if they were specifically linked with a central theme of mental disorder and only if they were presented as relating to a disorder.

Thus material was considered relevant and analyzed if it presented anything directly or indirectly related to mental illness. For example, material would be considered relevant if one of the characters in a drama were spoken of as "insane," if someone were being treated by a psychiatrist, if a person's behavior was called "emotionally disturbed," or if someone exhibited any of the classical neurotic symptoms. Whereas in a sense relevant material was defined rather narrowly (concerning mental disorders), the indicants of these disorders in media presentations were construed rather broadly. In some instances, it was very easy to determine the relevance of a presentation for the content analysis, for example, a newspaper story about "an escaped mental patient." In other cases, the decision of relevancy was debatable. In all cases, material was considered relevant and analyzed only if two out of three coders, working independently, rated the media excerpt as relevant. Because, as we found later, the occurrence of relevant material is much the exception rather than the rule, the odds that two out of three coders would rate an item relevant "by chance" were relatively low.

PRELIMINARY SCREENING FOR RELEVANCY.   Our first analysis was directed at television. There, relevance of material had to be judged immediately before the content-analysis procedures were applied. If the coder decided that the material was relevant, he marked it appropriately for content categories while the program was in progress. With radio programs, magazines, and newspapers, relevancy could be judged at any time before the content analysis was applied.

When we found that relevant material occurs relatively infrequently in television, we assumed that it would occur relatively infrequently in the other media as well. After inspection, much of the material could be discarded as clearly irrelevant (such as financial reports of civic organizations, most advertisements, articles about club meetings, weather maps, and musical programs). Thus, to reduce the work load, the original plan of having three coders judge the relevance of *every* media presentation was discarded in favor of a plan whereby only one coder would judge content relevancy in a preliminary screening. Material that was in no wise related could be thrown out in that screening. Then three coders would work over the reduced collection of material, and the final judgment of relevancy would be based, as before, on majority decision.

CONTENT-ANALYSIS RESULTS

How seriously can the results of the content analysis be taken? We have pointed out some of the frailties of the procedures that were used. Much of the data is judgmental and is no better or no worse than the subjective processes of the coders. Also, the content samples were, at best, only moderately representative of the media as a whole. In spite of the limitations of the content analysis and the modest proportions of our media samples, however, the results are so lopsided that we can reach some strong conclusions about the mental-health content of the mass media.

Time and Space

Seeking material directly related to mental-health problems (as we defined them) in the mass media is like looking for a needle in a haystack. If you search every inch of space in three different daily newspapers, the odds are that you will find only one item which is relevant. To find one relevant item it would be necessary to read, on the average, the entire content of two magazines. If you listened to one entire day of broadcasting of a radio station, you would, on the average, find about 2.3 programs with information or portrayals relevant to mental-health problems. An almost identical number of relevant programs would be expected in the entire daily telecasting of one station—2.4 programs which in some way relate to mental-health problems. Thus we can conclude that:

PROPOSITION 1: *Information concerning mental illness appears relatively infrequently in mass-media presentations.*

The findings here contradict our original estimates of the prevalence of mental-health presentations in the mass media. We had guessed that relevant material was presented more frequently than it is. Before doing the study we tried to recall the number of presentations relating to mental-health issues that we had seen recently in newspapers, television, and the other media, but in so doing we did not fully consider the many programs that were irrelevant. Consequently, we overestimated, percentagewise, the occurrence of related material.

In all of the media samples combined, we found a total of 202 relevant items (items being defined as separate whole programs in radio and television and as columns, stories, and features in the printed media). Of the total, we found 120 items in newspapers, 49 in magazines, 16 in radio, and 17 in television. There were not enough items for us to compare their content similarities and differences or to demonstrate differences among subclassifications of the media. For example, it would have been interesting to determine whether the mental-health content of newspapers is generally different from that of television programs or whether the mental-health content of television news programs is different from that of evening drama programs. Because there were not enough relevant items to analyze separately, all of the relevant material was lumped together, providing an average profile of the information presented in the mass media.

Although we did not study the issue directly, it seemed to us that information relating to "physical" disorders—cancer, heart trouble, physical injury, and so forth—appeared more frequently than information relating to mental health. Perhaps the apparent relative scarcity of information relevant to mental-health problems is related to the findings that public information is unstructured and uncrystallized. Problems of mental health may not be discussed sufficiently in the media, in schools, and in private conversation to permit the individual to develop a firm system of beliefs. More research is needed, however, to determine the amount of mental-health information in the media and, if, as our data indicate, such information is relatively scarce, to test the effect of this scarcity on public beliefs.

The Information Factors

To review: Two out of three coders had to be in agreement before material was classed as relevant and before content was coded on the information factors. Although basing the analysis on majority decisions reduced the total amount of data, it probably produced a more valid set of results.

While the data on the information held by the public and the experts was in seven-step-scale form and could be compared directly, the data from this content analysis had to be converted to the seven-step scale for comparison purposes. The data consisted of ratings by coders of the number of times that one pole of a factor was portrayed as compared with the other pole. For example, 80 instances were found in which the "immediate external environment" (Factor VII) was portrayed as being at the root of particular mental disorders. The opposite pole of the factor, "personality dynamics," was portrayed only 29 times. Thus Factor VII was attributed to be the cause in 73 percent of the classified presentations. Percentages of this kind were then converted to a seven-point scale (see Nunnally, 1957, for a description

of the scaling procedure used). From these converted results
we were able to compare the results from the mass media
with the opinions held by the public and the experts (see
Fig. 3.1).

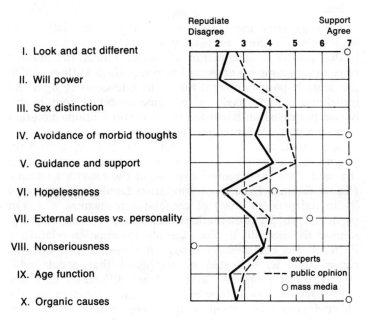

FIGURE 3.1   Comparisons of Experts, the Public, and the Mass Media
on the Ten Information Factors

The scaled factor scores for the media, represented by
circles, are shown in Figure 3.1. Three factors (will power,
sex distinction, and age function) occurred less than ten
times in the media presentations and consequently offered
insufficient grounds for making comparisons. The factor
scores for the media are compared with the average responses given by experts and by members of the general
public. . . . The results are quite clear. Not only are the views
that the media present generally incorrect according to expert

opinion but they are also far less accurate than the beliefs of the average man.

PROPOSITION 2: *The media of mass communication generally present a distorted picture of mental-health problems.*

Although some mass-media presentations, especially those specifically designed to convey information about mental health, provide a valid picture of mental illness, the number of such programs is very small in comparison to those which incidentally portray mental illness in a misleading light. An individual is more likely to see some aspect of neurotic behavior portrayed on television in an evening drama program than in a public-information program.

In general, the causes, symptoms, methods of treatment, prognoses, and social effects of mental illness portrayed by the media are far removed from what the experts advocate. (These findings from the information factors are supported by an independent study of confession magazines. . . . (In particular, media presentations emphasize the bizarre symptoms of the mentally ill. For example, information relating to Factor I was recorded 89 times. Of these, 88 affirmed the factor, that is, indicated or suggested that people with mental-health problems "look and act different"; only one item denied Factor I. In television dramas, for example, the afflicted person often enters the scene staring glassy-eyed, with his mouth widely agape, mumbling incoherent phrases or laughing uncontrollably. Even in what would be considered the milder disorders, neurotic phobias and obsessions, the afflicted person is presented as having bizarre facial expressions and actions.

The occurrence of mental disorder is explained in the media most often by pressures in the immediate external environment (Factor VII). The soap-opera heroine develops a neurosis because her husband dies in a plane crash, her little daughter is afflicted with an incurable disease, and all the family savings are lost in a fire. The "neurosis" goes away with a brighter turn of events. If the pressures of the immediate external environment are not brought in as causal explanations, organic factors are cited. A magazine fiction story might explain neurotic or psychotic behavior in terms of an old battlefield injury, a head wound in childhood, or physical privation such as thirst or hunger.

In the media, the person with a mental disorder most often receives help from some strong person in the environment who lends guidance and support. The strong individual may be a person who is professionally trained—a psychiatrist, "doctor," or nurse; equally often the guiding hand is that of a homespun philosopher who manages to say the right thing at the right time. Such cogencies as "The world is what you make of it" and "The past cannot hurt you" are portrayed as profoundly influencing the course of a disorder.

Supplementary Categories

Because only a few examples of the items in the media contained material which was related to the supplementary categories, there is little to report. For example, in the category "whom to seek for advice," we found that only eight psychiatrists, two "doctors," one psychologist, and one nurse were mentioned. These categories did provide one interesting bit of negative evidence: Although we had thought that the media might portray religion as being related to mental-health issues, it was seldom mentioned as an important variable. The same results held in a separate study of confession magazines. In this case, the media are in line with public opinion: our studies show that very few people associate mental-health phenomena with religion.

Attitude Ratings

The media samples portrayed 41 persons who could be classified as mentally ill. Of these, 21 displayed typical neurotic symptoms and 20 displayed typical psychotic symptoms. Three coders made attitude ratings of the 41 portrayals, and the median rating of the three coders on each Semantic Differential scale was used in the analysis. The resulting profile of the mentally ill in the mass media closely resembles the public's attitudes toward the mentally ill. Both psychotics and neurotics are portrayed as relatively ignorant, dangerous, dirty, unkind, and unpredictable. Neurotics were pictured as less dangerous, dirty, and unkind than psychotics, the latter being pictured as stronger and more active.

For what they are worth, the coders also made attitude ratings of the portrayals of the 12 "therapists" mentioned above. The resulting average profile is much the same as the attitude profile of the general public toward psychologists and psychiatrists. The media portrayals depict the therapist as being intelligent, kind, and valuable.

SUMMARY

Our results point to a seeming paradox: the ideas about mental health portrayed in the mass media are less "correct" in comparison to expert opinion than are the beliefs of the public at large. Where then did the public get its present body of information? Certainly not from an uncritical acceptance of media presentations. Perhaps, as has been suggested, the public is able to discriminate between "valid" information and unrealistic portrayals. If this is so, then the public probably does learn something from the "better" media presentations, although the number of such programs is relatively small.

The media are, of course, commercial ventures whose policies and presentations are determined in part by their internal needs. Presentations related to mental health are shaped by numerous hands—writers, editors, directors, media executives, commercial sponsors, and others. Perhaps it is necessary to emphasize bizarre symptoms in order to make the presentations more exciting and to enlarge their audience appeal. Perhaps the relatively restricted time period or space available is responsible for much of the oversimplified treatment of mental disorders. If the media took the time to illustrate the complexities of the learning processes that experts deem to be the important components in personality disorders, they might produce some very dull programs.

The communications media have adopted a stylized picture of mental-health problems which distorts reality, but is a useful device in drama, comedy, and other programs for the public. It would be a great waste, however, if the communications media did not eventually help to promote a healthy set of public attitudes and improve public understanding of mental-health phenomena. It is also to be hoped that more accurate information can be incorporated into effective forms of entertainment. Our content analysis was performed in 1954 and 1955. Presentations in the mass media may have begun to incorporate more adequate viewpoints about mental health since then.

Rejection: A Possible Consequence of Seeking Help for Mental Disorders

DEREK L. PHILLIPS

The nonconformist, whether he be foreigner or "odd ball," intellectual or idiot, genius or jester, individualist or hobo, physically or mentally abnormal—pays a price for "being different" unless his peculiarity is considered acceptable for his particular group, or unless he lives in a place or period of particularly high tolerance or enlightenment.[1]

The penalty that *mentally ill* persons pay for "being different" is often rejection by others in the community. Following the increased interest of social scientists in the public's attitudes toward the mentally ill,[2] this research investigates some of the factors involved in the rejection of mentally ill individuals.

FROM the *American Sociological Review* 28 (December, 1963) 963–972. Reprinted by permission of the author and publisher. This investigation was carried out during the tenure of a Predoctoral Fellowship from the National Institute of Mental Health. The writer wishes to thank C. Richard Fletcher, Phillip S. Hammond, and Elton F. Jackson for their helpful suggestions.

This paper presents the results of a controlled experiment in influencing people's attitudes toward individuals exhibiting symptoms of mental illness. The research attempts to determine the extent to which people's attitudes toward an individual exhibiting disturbed behavior are related to their knowledge of the particular help-source that the individual is using or has used. The term "help-source" here refers to such community resources as clergymen, physicians, psychiatrists, marriage counselors, mental hygiene clinics, alcohol clinics, and mental hospitals, each of which is frequently concerned with persons having emotional problems.

Most studies concerned with attitudes toward the mentally ill have focused on the individual's behavior as the sole factor determining whether or not he is rejected by others. Other research has considered the importance of psychiatric treatment or hospitalization in *identifying* the individual as mentally ill and, subsequently, leading to his rejection.[3] But as far as could be determined, no study has been made of the importance of utilizing other help-sources in determining or influencing public attitudes toward individuals exhibiting disturbed behavior.

In a number of studies respondents have been asked whether they considered various *descriptions* to be those of mentally ill persons, and some respondents were found unable to recognize certain serious symptoms of disturbed behavior. Star, for example, asking 3500 respondents about six case abstracts of mentally ill persons, found that 17 percent of the sample said that none of these imaginary persons was sufficiently deviant to represent what they meant by mental illness. Another 28 percent limited their concept of mental illness to the paranoid, the only description where violence was a prominent feature of the behavior.[4] Elaine and John Cumming, asking questions about the same six descriptions of deviant behavior, found that the majority of people dismissed the descriptions, even when they were clinically grave, as normal, with such comments as "It's just a quirk, it's nothing serious."[5]

Sharply in disagreement with these findings, however, are the results of studies by Lemkau and Crocetti, and by Dohrenwend, Bernard, and Kolb. Using three of the Star abstracts, Lemkau and Crocetti found that 91 percent of their sample identified the paranoid as mentally ill, 78 percent identified the simple schizophrenic, and 62 percent identified the alcoholic.[6] Dohrenwend and his associates, interviewing "leaders in an urban area," used the six Star abstracts. They report that "all saw mental illness in the description of paranoid schizophrenia; 72 percent saw it in the example of simple schizophrenia; 63 percent in the alcoholic; about 50 percent in the anxiety neurosis and in the juvenile character disorder; and 40 percent in the compulsive-phobic."[7] These findings, although somewhat inconsistent, do indicate some public ignorance concerning the signs and symptoms of mental illness. More important here, they tell us nothing about how the public *feels* toward the individuals in these case abstracts.

Hospitalization is another cue that has been found to influence recognition of a person as mentally ill. The Cummings state, "Mental illness, it seems, is a condition which afflicts people who must go to a mental institution, but up until they go almost anything they do is fairly normal."[8]

Apparently some people can correctly identify symptoms of mental illness and others cannot, while for some the mentally ill are only those who have been in a mental hospital. But it seems equally important to ask whether people *reject* individuals displaying symptoms of mental illness or those who have been hospitalized. In part, the task of this research was to determine the extent to which people reject various descriptions of disturbed behavior. An additional cue—the *help-source* that the individual described is utilizing —was presented to the respondents in order to ascertain the importance of the help-source in determining rejection of mentally ill individuals. Four help-sources that people with mental disorders often consult[9]—the clergyman, the physician, the psychiatrist, and the mental hospital—were represented.

Several recent studies have been concerned with the help-sources that people suggest using for mental disorders, as well as the ones they actually have used.[10] Considerable evidence from these studies indicates that people have strong negative attitudes toward psychiatrists and mental hospitals and toward individuals using either of these help-sources.[11] But there seems to be no evidence of negative attitudes toward clergymen or physicians, or toward people consulting these two help-sources. Further, the fact that people with emotional problems are more likely to consult clergymen and physicians than psychiatrists and mental hospitals[12] suggests the absence of strong negative attitudes toward the latter and those utilizing them. Gurin points out that they ". . . are the areas most people turn to with their personal problems; they are the major "gatekeepers" in the treatment process, either doing the treating themselves or referring to a more specialized professional resource."[13] Both the clergyman and the physician are professionally involved in what are usually defined as "the private affairs" of others. They have, what Naegele calls ". . . legitimate access to realms beyond public discussion."[14]

Although it is probably true that the public does not hold negative attitudes toward clergymen and physicians, I suggest that an individual consulting either of these help-sources may more often lose face, and more often be regarded as deviant, than an individual exhibiting the same behavior who does not consult one of these professional resources. How does this come to be so?

As Clausen and Yarrow point out, "There is an ethic of being able to handle one's own problems by oneself, which applies not only to psychiatric problems."[15] Similarly, Ewalt says, "One value in American culture compatible with most approaches to a definition of positive mental health appears to be this: An individual should be able to stand on his own two feet without making undue demands or impositions on others."[16] In another statement of this view, Kadushin reports that, in answer to the question "Would you tell people in general that you came here?" (the Peale-Blanton Religio-Psychiatric Clinic), a respondent replied ". . . I wouldn't tell people in general. I know that there's still a stigma attached to people who seek psychiatric aid, and I guess I'm ashamed that I couldn't manage my own problem."[17]

Thus, an outside observer's knowledge that a person is consulting any of the four help-sources discussed may have at least two important consequences for the individual with a behavior problem: (1) He is defined as someone who *has* a problem. Moreover, the further along the continuum from clergyman to mental hospital the individual moves, the more his problem is seen as a serious one, and individuals consulting a psychiatrist or a mental hospital are very often defined as "mentally ill" or "insane." (2) The individual is defined as unable to handle his problem by himself.

I am suggesting that the reported inability of some persons to recognize certain serious symptoms of disturbed behavior is due to difficulty in evaluating an individual's behavior, and that knowledge about what help-source the individual is utilizing helps others decide whether he is "deviant" or has a problem that he cannot cope with himself. And an important social consequence for the person who, because of his behavior or choice of help-source, is defined as deviant may be *rejection.*

These considerations led to formulation of the following hypothesis: Individuals exhibiting identical behavior will be increasingly rejected as they are described as not seeking any help, as utilizing a clergyman, a physician, a psychiatrist, or a mental hospital.

METHOD

To test this hypothesis, interviews were conducted with a systematic sample[18] of 300 married white females selected from the address section of the City Directory of Branford, a southern New England town of approximately 17,000 population.[19] The sample was so small that the need to control for a number of variables was obvious. Thus, males,[20] non-whites, and unmarried respondents were excluded from the sample.

The interviews took place in the respondents' homes and were of 20 to 40 minutes duration. Each respondent was given five cards, one at a time, describing different behaviors. The interviewer read each description aloud from the interview schedule as the respondent followed by reading the card.

Case abstract (A) was a description of a paranoid schizophrenic, (B) an individual suffering from simple schizophrenia, (C) an anxious-depressed person, (D) a phobic individual with compulsive features, and (E) a "normal" person. The first four abstracts were, in the main, the same as those developed by Shirley Star, formerly of the National Opinion Research Center in Chicago.[21] The fifth abstract, that of the "normal"[22] individual, was developed expressly for this research.[23]

The five case abstracts were presented in combination with information about what help-source an individual was utilizing, in the following manner:

 1. Nothing was added to the description of the behavior —this was, of course, the absence of any help.

 2. Affixed to the description was the statement: "He has been going to see his clergyman regularly about the way he is getting along."

 3. Affixed to the description was the statement: "He has been going to see his physician regularly about the way he is getting along."

 4. Affixed to the description was the statement: "He has been going to see his psychiatrist regularly about the way he is getting along."

 5. Affixed to the description was the statement: "He has been in a mental hospital because of the way he was getting along."

This research required an experimental design permitting classification of each of the two independent variables (behavior and help-source) in five categories.[24] Observations for all possible combinations of the values of the two variables would have been desirable, but this clearly was not feasible. Hence the observations were arranged in the form of a Graeco-Latin Square[25] so as to obtain a large amount of information from a relatively small number of observations. Specifically, this type of design enables us to discover: (a) the influence of different types of behavior in determining rejection, and (b) the influence of different help-sources in determining rejection.

The 300 respondents were divided at random into five groups of 60 individuals each. Every individual in each group saw five combinations of behavior and help-source, but no group or individual saw any given behavior or any given help-source more than once. In order to assure that the rejection rates were not affected by the *order* in which individuals saw the combinations, the experiment was designed so that each behavior and each help-source was seen first by one group, second by another, third by another, fourth by another, and last by the remaining group.[26]

Thus, in the Graeco-Latin Square design, three variables were considered (behavior, help-source, and order). The data were classified in five categories on each of these variables. See Table 1, where the letters in each cell indicate a descrip-

TABLE 1.   The Graeco-Latin Square Design

| | \multicolumn{5}{c}{Order} | | | | |
	1	2	3	4	5
Group 1	A1	B2	C3	D4	E5
Group 2	B3	C4	D5	E1	A2
Group 3	C5	D1	E2	A3	B4
Group 4	D2	E3	A4	B5	C1
Group 5	E4	A5	B1	C2	D3

NOTE: N for each cell in the table is 60.

tion of behavior, and the numbers in each cell indicate the help-source utilized. In the top left-hand cell, for example, the letter A indicates that the paranoid schizophrenic was the description seen first by Group 1, and that he was described as seeing help-source 1 (that is, he was not described as seeking any help). Similarly, in the bottom right-hand cell, the letter D indicates that the phobic-compulsive person was the abstract seen fifth by Group 5, and that he was described as consulting help-source 3 (a physician).

After reading each combination of behavior and help-source, the respondents were asked a uniform series of questions. These questions made up a social distance scale, indicating how close a relation the respondent was willing to tolerate with the individuals in the case abstracts. This scale was used as the measure of *rejection*, the dependent variable in the research.

The social distance scale consisted of the following items:

(1) "Would you discourage your children from marrying someone like this?" (2) "If you had a room to rent in your home, would you be willing to rent it to someone like this?" (3) "Would you be willing to work on a job with someone like this?" (4) "Would you be willing to have someone like this join a favorite club or organization of yours?" (5) "Would you object to having a person like this as a neighbor?"[27]

The range of possible scores for each combination of help-source and behavior was from zero (when no items indicated rejection) through five (when all items indicated rejection). A test of reproducibility was applied and the resulting coefficient was .97, indicating that the scale met acceptable standards; i.e., was a unidimensional scale.

It should be emphasized that each combination of behavior and help-source was seen by 60 respondents. It also bears repeating that each respondent was presented with five combinations of behavior and help-source. Thus, each respondent contributed a rejection score (on the social distance scale) to each of 5 cells out of the 25 cells in Table 1. An analysis of variance of the form generally applied to planned experiments was carried out.[28]

RESULTS AND DISCUSSION

Table 2 presents the mean rejection rate for each combination of behavior and help-source. An individual exhibiting a given type of behavior is increasingly rejected as he is described as seeking no help, as seeing a clergyman, as seeing a physician, as seeing a psychiatrist, or as having been in a mental hospital. The relation between the independent variable (help-source) and the dependent variable (rejection) is statistically significant at the .001 level. Furthermore, the reversal in the "paranoid schizophrenic" row is the only one among 25 combinations.[29]

The relation between the other independent variable (behavior) and rejection is also significant at the .001 level. In fact, the F obtained for the relation between behavior and rejection (F = 64.52) is much higher than the F obtained for

TABLE 2. Rejection Scores[a] for Each Help-Source and Behavior Combination[b]

Behavior	Help-Source Utilized: No help	Clergy-man	Physician	Psychia-trist	Mental Hospital	Total
Paranoid schizophrenic	3.65	3.33	3.77	4.12	4.33	3.84
Simple schizophrenic	1.10	1.57	1.83	2.85	3.68	2.21
Depressed-neurotic	1.45	1.62	2.07	2.70	3.28	2.22
Phobic-compulsive	.53	1.12	1.18	1.87	2.27	1.39
Normal individual	.02	.22	.50	1.25	1.63	.72
TOTAL	1.35	1.57	1.87	2.56	3.04	—

NOTE: $F = 23.53$, $p < .001$

[a] Rejection scores are represented by the mean number of items rejected on the Social Distance Scale.

[b] N for each cell in the table is 60.

the relation between help-source and rejection ($F = 23.53$). In other words, when a respondent was confronted with a case abstract containing both a description of their individual's behavior and information about what help-source he was utilizing, the description of behavior played a greater part (i.e., accounted for more variance) than the help-source in determining how strongly she rejected the individual described.

As was indicated earlier, the main purpose of this presentation is to show the extent to which attitudes toward an individual exhibiting symptoms of mental illness are related to knowledge of the particular help-source that he is utilizing. The importance of the type of behavior is of secondary interest here; I have investigated the relation between behavior and rejection mainly to ascertain the *relative* importance of each of the two elements presented in the case abstracts. The relation between behavior and rejection will be fully treated in a future paper.

The totals at the bottom of Table 1 show that the largest

increase in the rejection rates occurs when an individual sees a psychiatrist. That is, the rejection rate for individuals described as consulting a physician (1.87) differs from the rejection rate for individuals described as consulting a psychiatrist (2.56) to a degree greater than for any other comparison between two adjacent help-sources. The second largest over-all increase in rejection occurs when the individual is described as having been in a mental hospital, and the smallest net increase (.20) occurs when the individual sees a clergyman, compared to seeking no help at all.

Probably the most significant aspect of the effect of help-source on rejection rates is that, for four of the five case abstracts, the biggest increase in rejection occurs when the individual is described as consulting a psychiatrist, and in three of the five abstracts the second largest increase occurs when the individual is depicted as having been in a mental hospital. Not only are individuals increasingly rejected as they are described as seeking no help, as seeing a clergyman, a physician, a psychiatrist, or a mental hospital, but they are *disproportionately* rejected when described as utilizing the latter two help-sources. This supports the suggestion made earlier that individuals utilizing psychiatrists and mental hospitals may be rejected not only because they have a health problem, and because they are unable to handle the problem themselves, but also because contact with a psychiatrist or a mental hospital defines them as "mentally ill" or "insane."

Despite the fact that the "normal" person is more an "ideal type" than a normal person, when he is described as having been in a mental hospital he is rejected more than a psychotic individual described as not seeking help or as seeing a clergyman, and more than a depressed-neurotic seeing a clergyman. Even when the normal person is described as seeing a psychiatrist, he is rejected more than a simple schizophrenic who seeks no help, more than a phobic-compulsive individual seeking no help or seeing a clergyman or physician.

As was noted previously, there is one reversal in Table 2. The paranoid schizophrenic, unlike the other descriptions, was rejected more strongly when he was described as not utilizing any help-source than when he was described as utilizing a clergyman. The paranoid was described in the case abstract as suspicious, as picking fights with people who did not even know him, and as cursing his wife. His behavior may be so threatening and so obviously deviates from normal behavior, that the respondents feel that he is socially less objectionable when he takes a step to help himself. In other words, the individual *obviously* in need of professional help is in a sense "rewarded" for seeking at least one kind of help, that of the clergyman. And though the paranoid schizophrenic is increasingly rejected when he is described as utilizing a physician, a psychiatrist, and a mental hospital, the relative amount of increase is much less than for the other four case abstracts.

Mentally ill persons whose behavior does not deviate markedly from normal role-expectations may be assigned responsibility for their own behavior. If so, seeking any professional help is an admission of inability to meet this responsibility. An individual whose behavior is markedly abnormal (in this instance, the paranoid schizophrenic) may not, however, be considered responsible for his behavior or for his recovery, and is, therefore, rejected less than other individuals when he seeks professional help.

CONTROLS

To determine whether the findings were spurious, the relation between help-source and rejection was observed under several different controls. The association was maintained within age groups, within religious affiliation groups, within educational attainment groups, and within groups occupying different positions in the status hierarchy.[30] The association was also maintained within groups differing in authoritarianism.[31]

But when (1) experience with someone who had sought help for emotional problems[32] and (2) attitude toward the norm of self-reliance,[33] were controlled, the relation between help-source and rejection was specified.

Table 3 presents the rejection rates for respondents reporting a relative who sought help, those reporting a friend who

TABLE 3.   Rejection Scores[a] for All Cases by Help-Source
and Acquaintance with Help-Seekers

Help-Source Utilized	Acquaintance		
	Relative (N=37)	Friend (N=73)	No one (N=190)
No help-source	2.35	1.45	1.12
Clergyman	2.06	1.45	1.51
Physician	1.30	1.58	2.09
Psychiatrist	2.08	2.53	2.66
Mental hospital	2.38	2.82	3.25

[a] Rejection scores are represented by the mean number of
items rejected on the Social Distance Scale.

sought help, and those who knew no one who sought help
for emotional problems. For ease of presentation and interpretation, the rejection rates for the five case abstracts have
been combined.[34]

There are two points of interest in Table 3. One is the
difference in rejection rates *among* the three groups of
respondents. But because these interesting differences are
peripheral to the central concern here, I will focus, instead,
on the second point of interest. This is the consistent increase
—*within* two of the three groups of respondents—in rejection
scores for persons not seeking any help, utilizing a clergyman, a physician, a psychiatrist, or a mental hospital.

Respondents *not* acquainted with a help-seeker as well as
those acquainted with a help-seeking *friend* adhere to the
pattern of rejection previously demonstrated in Table 2. But
respondents with a help-seeking *relative* deviate markedly
from this pattern. They reject persons not seeking help more
than they do persons consulting a clergyman, physician, or
psychiatrist, and almost as much as those utilizing a mental
hospital. And they reject persons consulting a clergyman
more than those consulting a physician.

Perhaps respondents with help-seeking relatives are more
able to recognize the behavior in the abstracts as that of
persons who *need* help and therefore they reject them
strongly when they do not seek help. A similar explanation

may apply to the rejection of persons using a clergyman. That is, these respondents may see the clergyman as not being what Parsons calls "technically competent help"[35] and equate seeing him with not seeking help. The comparatively low rejection of persons consulting a physician may reflect the respondents' belief that a physician is one of the professional resources that one *should* utilize for emotional problems, and that a physician brings the least stigma to the user; whereas the psychiatrist and the mental hospital, though both competent resources, tend to stigmatize the user much more.[36]

The reader will recall that one of the case abstracts presented to the respondents was that of a "normal" individual. Since respondents with a help-seeking relative may reject the non-help-seeking cases because they are recognized as needing help, including the description of the normal person may "distort" the findings. The rejection rates for the four mentally ill abstracts have, therefore, been separated from those for the normal person and presented in Table 4. In-

TABLE 4. Rejection Scores[a] for All Mentally Ill Cases by Help-Source and Acquaintance with Help-Seekers

| Help-Source Utilized | Acquaintance | | |
	Relative (N=37)	Friend (N=73)	No one (N = 190)
No help-source	2.81	1.64	1.16
Clergyman	2.20	1.65	1.86
Physician	1.51	1.91	2.46
Psychiatrist	2.45	2.88	2.90
Mental hospital	3.04	3.14	3.51

[a] Rejection scores are represented by the mean number of items rejected on the Social Distance Scale.

spection of this table reveals the same pattern found in Table 2, except that the rejection rate for persons utilizing each help-source is somewhat higher than in Table 3.[37]

Turning now to the relation between adherence to the norm of self-reliance and rejection of persons described as using the various help-sources, the data in Table 5 indicate that the association between help-source and rejection is maintained even among those who do not strongly adhere to the norm of self-reliance.[38] Among respondents agreeing either strongly or somewhat to the norm of self-reliance there is a consistent increase in rejection of persons as they moved from no help to the mental hospital. Respondents *not* adhering to the norm of self-reliance, however, reject persons not seeking help more than they do persons seeing a clergyman or a physician.[39]

TABLE 5.   Rejection Scores[a] for All Cases by Help-Source and Adherence to the Norm of Self-Reliance

Help-Source Utilized	Adherence to Norm of Self-Reliance		
	Disagree (N=28)	Agree Somewhat (N=128)	Agree Strongly (N=144)
No help-source	1.79	1.39	1.22
Clergyman	1.68	1.56	1.52
Physician	1.67	1.87	2.00
Psychiatrist	2.43	2.52	2.65
Mental hospital	2.64	3.09	3.23

[a] Rejection scores are represented by the mean number of items rejected on the Social Distance Scale.

This pattern is similar to the one followed by respondents who had help-seeking relatives (see Table 3),[40] and the same general interpretation may be appropriate. Respondents who do not agree that people should handle their own problems may view people seeing a clergyman as "handling their own problems." If this is true, then those not adhering to the norm of self-reliance would be expected to reject persons who see a clergyman, as well as those who seek no help.

Thus, for the great majority of respondents, who either (1) have not had experience with a relative who sought help for emotional problems, or (2) adhere to the norm of self-reliance, help-source and rejection are strongly associated.[41]

On the other hand, respondents who have had experience

with a help-seeking relative deviate quite sharply from the rejection pattern of the majority, as do those who do not adhere to the norm of self-reliance. Nevertheless, this deviant pattern appears to make sense theoretically. Those acquainted with a help-seeking relative, having had more exposure to sick-role prescriptions, may be highly rejecting of persons not seeking help because they feel that people should seek "technically competent help." Respondents not adhering to the norm of self-reliance may reject non-help-seekers for a similar reason. They too may feel that handling one's own problems is inappropriate, and that people should seek competent help. And, as suggested previously, both groups may equate help from a clergyman with no help at all.[42]

CONCLUSIONS AND IMPLICATIONS

On the basis of these findings from a southern New England town, the source of help sought by mentally disturbed individuals appears to be strongly related to the degree to which others in the community reject them. Individuals are increasingly rejected as they are described as utilizing no help, as utilizing a clergyman, a physician, a psychiatrist, or a mental hospital.

Controls for age, religion, education, social class, and authoritarianism failed to diminish the relationship, but controls for experience with an emotionally disturbed help-seeker and for adherence to the norm of self-reliance tended to specify it. Respondents who had had experience with a help-seeking relative deviated markedly from the pattern followed by the rest of the sample, as did respondents not adhering to the norm of self-reliance. Both of these groups rejected people seeking no help more than they did those consulting a clergyman or a physician, and respondents with help-seeking relatives also reject non-help-seekers more than those consulting a psychiatrist. Both groups rejected persons seeing a clergyman more than those seeing a physician.

The evidence presented here suggests that a mentally ill person who seeks help may be rejected by others in the community. The findings also have implications for what

Mechanic and Volkart call "the inclination to adopt the sick role."[43] We can easily imagine an individual who, because he fears the stigma attached to the help-seeker, does not utilize a professional resource for his problems. Avoiding the possibility of rejection, he also denies himself technically competent help.[44]

Thus the utilization of certain help-sources involves not only a *reward* (positive mental health), but also a *cost* (rejection by others and, consequently, a negative self-image);[45] we need to assess the net balance of gains and losses resulting from seeking help for problems of disturbed behavior.

The present analysis has been concerned with the rejection of help-seekers in hypothetical situations. Future research should be designed so that it would be possible to examine the rejection of help-seekers in "real" situations. Hopefully, the present research will provide some understanding and raise significant questions about the consequences of seeking help for problems of disturbed behavior in our society.

Look At Me

PETER GREY

The Minnesota State Hospital stood on a hill to the north of Fergus Falls. It was not such a great hill as to permit the asylum buildings to loom over the town; you could not see them from any of the downtown streets, or even from the courthouse steeple. But in the country, out on the prairie, looking back from a few miles away, you could see only the

FROM "The New Yorker," March 23, 1963, 133–143. Reprinted by permission of the author and the publisher.

immense, impersonal asylum on the landscape, and nothing
of the town itself, with its church spires, its broom factory
and casket factory, nesting in the sheltered valley. It is over
a distance of many years that I now look back to the prominence of the madhouse in the panorama of my childhood in
Fergus.

Lester Nelson, Herbert Johnson, and I sometimes went to
the Great Northern Station at a quarter to five in the afternoon to see the train come in from Minneapolis, bringing
perhaps two or three travelling salesmen in city clothes, and
now and then a nurse in charge of an insane woman in a
funny hat, or of several insane women in funny hats. The
nurse would shepherd her charges across the platform and
into the asylum's horse-drawn station wagon, which had two
lengthwise seats and was boxed with thick wire netting like
a cage. Invariably, these women presented a dishevelled or
ruffled appearance, like so many sick turkeys—a torn blouse,
a petticoat or a black stocking coming down, a shoe unlaced,
hair uncombed or flying wild, and a disorder in the eyes.
Sometimes a male attendant would get off the train with his
unshaven, dishevelled charges. Though less dishevelled than
the women, because of the simpler nature of men's clothing,
they also wore funny headgear—a hunting cap with dangling
ear flaps, a red stocking cap, a caved-in derby. I remember
once seeing two poor men leave the train in strait jackets,
with heads bare and faces bruised. I knew very well it was
bad manners to gawk, but I gawked anyway as they went
shuffling, gliding, shambling across the platform to the cage
on wheels. Occasionally one of them would take exuberant
steps, as in a crazy dance, and the next day Lester and
Herbert and I would make each other laugh by walking
crazy. "Look at me. I'm that old loony."

There were other afternoons when the three of us bicycled
up the asylum hill and on the cinder driveways around the
many buildings. We would pedal slowly past the immense,
netted, open-air porches, inside which figures paced back and
forth, back and forth, and we would go slowly past the other
figures seated on the lawns. As a rule, the figures on the
grass, each at a lonely distance from the others, did not raise
their heads to glance at us riding by, or at anything. We

would pass a few animated figures also—a man chasing grasshoppers, a woman revolving like a dervish, a gaunt fellow waving a green branch and cawing at passersby. Almost always we would see at least one worth mimicking afterward. "Look. I'm that old loony."

Unlike several of our friends, Lester, Herbert, and I had no family connections with the asylum. But from the boys whose parents, aunts, or uncles were employed there in some such capacity as nurse, guard, or cook, we heard accounts of the life inside, particularly accounts of violence—a doctor stabbed with a kitchen knife, a stampede of thirty patients in a ward, a suicide by hanging. (This last was described so forcefully that the picture sank into my imagination to reappear in nightmares.) We also heard stories of escaped patients. I do not know whether these stories were true or made up, like ghost stories. Mrs. A. J. Comstock, so I heard, once opened her bedroom closet door to take out some article of clothing and put her hand on the bearded face of a lunatic hiding there among her summer dresses. Soren Rasmusson, according to another story, found a runaway from the asylum asleep in the haymow of his barn. The fellow had been hiding around there for a week, eating raw eggs from the henhouse and carrots from the garden. Someone else discovered, in the potato bin of his cellar, a runaway who nearly strangled him.

These stories seemed true, more than true, at the time; they peopled the recesses of the night for me. The unlighted back stairs at home became impossible in the evening, and for a while I felt compelled to look under my bed before going to sleep. But fear has its pleasurable side as well. It added a fierce thrill to hide-and-seek, kick-the-can, and our other hiding games. "Let's play it crazy," we would say. "We'll be run-away loonies, and the one who's 'it' will be the guard." "Playing it crazy" meant running wildly, screaming like mad, hiding in impossible places, and then going home still in a fever of excitement, which would have to be dissembled. On going into the house (after first wiping my shoes on the mat, and being careful not to let any flies in or the screen door bang) I would walk with circumspection, speak in a modulated voice, and wash my face and hands for supper.

One evening, my father, a deacon in the Congregational Church, announced across the supper table to my mother that he had invited a Mr. Larkin to have Sunday dinner with us. My great-grandmother, who lived with us, and I pricked up our ears.

"Tomorrow is Friday," said Mother, "and I had planned to bake a batch of bread. But now all the curtains in the front rooms will have to be washed and stretched. Perhaps I could get Mrs. Knudson to come in and give me a hand."

"You won't have to go to any extra trouble because of Mr. Larkin," said my father.

"Also, the silver needs to be polished, and the pictures in the front rooms should be taken down and cleaned," Mother went on. "Last time, Consuelo put them back all crooked, and when I remonstrated with her she said they'd straighten themselves out in a day or two."

"Mr. Larkin won't notice whether the curtains have been washed recently or not, or the condition of the silver, or the dust on the pictures," my father said.

"But *I* shall. Perhaps both Mrs. Knudson and Mrs. Schuck could come in to give me a hand."

"One of your regular Sunday dinners, without any fuss, my dear," said Father.

"I can't say I ever knew any Larkins," said Grandma Ah-Ah. (When no grownups were around, my cousins and I referred to our great-grandmother by that name because she would silently come into a room and cry "Ah-Ah!" at whoever was slouching or giggling or about to touch something he shouldn't, such as the stuffed owl in Aunt Annie Laurie's house, or my father's telescope. "Ah-Ah!" was all she had to say to make you freeze.)

"Yes, who is this Mr. Larkin?" asked Mother.

"The younger brother of a Miss Larkin I once knew in Madison," said Father.

"This is the first I've heard of your Miss Larkin in Madison," said Mother.

"Miss Larkin is now Mrs. Osgood. She has written asking me to find out how her brother is getting along. So this afternoon I went to see him, and I had a talk with Dr. Dorken."

"Dr. Dorken of the asylum? You went to the asylum to see Mr. Larkin? Is Mr. Larkin . . .?"

Father nodded. "Dr. Dorken agreed it might be of benefit to Mr. Larkin to come here for Sunday dinner. A change of scene, you understand."

"I shall bake an angel-food cake," said Mother. "And I shall certainly have the curtains washed and the pictures down for a cleaning."

"I've known mad people before in my day," said Grandma Ah-Ah. "The thing to do is to keep them diverted."

This was an unusually long speech for Grandma Ah-Ah to make, and it was unusual also for her to pay attention to general conversation. As a rule, she heard only what was addressed directly to her, and she would respond with a word or two, or not at all. Occasionally she had what my mother called "difficult days," when her mind became confused. Her real name was Grandmother Folsom; she was my mother's grandmother, and very old. She always sat very straight in her chair, and she smelled of lavender bags.

"Were they Indians, Grandma?" I asked.

"Eh?"

"All those mad people you used to know, were they Indians?"

"One was."

"What'd he do, Grandma?"

"Children should be seen, not heard," she said. It was an old voice coming to you from before you were born, coming hoarse through a prairie fire and a drought and a flood and hard winters and Indian trouble. All her life Grandma Ah-Ah had opposed slovenliness and uncleanliness and wickedness.

After supper, I asked my parents about Mr. Larkin. Would he come to our house with a guard? In a strait jacket? What would we do if he started to stab somebody or run away and hide? Father said my main problem would be how to be a good boy; I might give that more thought. Mother said I had better go to the kitchen and dry the supper dishes for Consuelo. "And it's quite unnecessary for you to say anything to Consuelo about Mr. Larkin. No need to put any more notions into her head."

I never knew in what mood I would find Consuelo—silent

and morose, eager for my company, antagonistic, or what. Sometimes she sang Spanish songs, sometimes Sunday-school hymns in English. What I liked best was her talk of Puerto Rico, where an uncle of mine, a missionary, had made a convert of her to the Presbyterian Church, and his wife, Aunt Minnehaha, had given her English lessons. Consuelo's talk, however, was of the time before her conversion; it was of cockfights and fiestas and the young men who had been in love with her. Every night and all night long, a man she'd never spoken to had stood across the street looking up at her window.

"Every single night, Consuelo?"

"Every single night."

"How long? For a month?"

"Every single night for two whole years. He was shy."

Or she would talk of the dances. Before going to a dance, she would pin fireflies in her hair, she said. Once, she made a crown of fireflies that everyone admired; she wore fragrant flowers at her waist, and always a fan on a long string of beads around her neck. She would sigh profoundly, thinking of those dances. I would look at her thick, kinky hair, which she combed once a month, and try to imagine her with the crown of fireflies. Three or four times, when we were certain Mother was in some distant part of the house, she tried to teach me to dance, there in the kitchen, while the dishwater cooled.

"What did the shy man do those nights you went to dances, Consuelo?" I once asked.

"I don't know. He was always there looking up at my window when I came back."

"But why did he look up at your window?"

"Because . . . Well, in Puerto Rico it's different. It's not like Fergus Falls."

Both Mrs. Knudson and Mrs. Schuck came that Friday and Saturday to wash and stretch curtains, polish the floors and the silver, and help with the baking. Saturday morning, just as I was about to go outdoors to play, Mother enlisted me to help chase flies out of the house. She gave us all—Mrs. Knudson, Mrs. Schuck, Consuelo, and me—copies of the Fergus Falls *Journal* to flap. We began in the kitchen, where the shades had been drawn, with Mother in the lead, rustling and flapping *Journals* in both hands, crying "Shoo, shoo!" and chasing two or three flies into the dining room. Then that door was closed, the dining-room shades were drawn to the sills, and all the flies were chased before us into the sitting room and parlor and eventually out the front door.

I decided not to tell Lester and Herbert that Mr. Larkin was coming to our house for Sunday dinner. Afterward I would tell them all about the visit, perhaps even act it out for them. "Look. I'm that old loony Larkin that came to our house." Neither Lester nor Herbert had ever met a loony. "Look at me," I would say.

Saturday afternoon, when Lester and Herbert and some other boys were playing croquet in the Johnsons' back yard, Mother sent me to mow our front and side lawns, though they had been mowed only a few days before. All day, she rustled through the downstairs rooms supervising the cleaning and occasionally taking a hand at it herself. She alone was permitted to touch Father's telescope. Consuelo and I and my three-year-old brother Phillip had been warned not even to go near the corner by the piano, where it rested on its tripod. It was Mother who dusted the telescope, and she performed this act with a solemnity suitable to an acolyte handling a sacred object. Yet she was no devotee of its mystery. On nights when Father had the telescope outdoors, he sometimes sent for her to share his view of the moon or some planet, and she would give a little peck of a glance through the tube. "Yes, it's very nice," she would say, and return to the house and her own familiar world. She, who used the word "my" many times oftener than Father, loved her family, her house, and her garden, and seemed to resent whatever was distant or alien. Why waste her time on the moon?

Father, on the other hand, was fascinated by the moon, I do believe because of its very inaccessibility. He gave to famine relief in China and missions in Africa because China and Africa were so far from Fergus Falls. He read the Bible and Homer and ancient history, and enjoyed speculation on what humanity would be like a thousand years hence. He took no interest in county elections or local gossip. He never worked in the garden, as Mother did; he would often stand at a distance from the garden, his gaze resting on the corn or the peas or the two flowering crabapple trees, in a state of abstraction. "I like to see things grow," he said. But not close up. That spoiled the view.

That Sunday, Mother and I were late to church because she still had so much to do to get the house ready for Mr. Larkin and to get the dinner started. Father had gone earlier, ahead of us. Grandma Ah-Ah never went to church any more; she could pray at home, she said. Consuelo had to miss both church and Sunday school that day, though she loved pipe-organ music and was a regular member of the Sunday-school choir. After church service was over, Mother hurried home, and I stayed on for Sunday school. Father drove the family horse and surrey straight from church to the asylum.

I was building block towers on the sitting-room floor for Phillip to knock down, when the doorbell rang and Mother came rustling in from the kitchen, her face flushed and a startled look in her eyes, to greet Mr. Larkin. At first sight, he was a disappointment—a clean-shaven, neat little man in a dark-gray suit, holding a derby like Father's. He thanked Mother for her welcome, and said he was pleased to be there. He smiled as if he was very pleased indeed. Yet there was a timidity about him, or a misgiving. For a while, it seemed as if he had to stay close to Father, with whom he was already acquainted. As he moved about the parlor and sitting room, he had to touch things—the door jamb, the wall, a tabletop, the back of a chair—as a blind person does, re-assuring himself through his fingertips. His gaze was keen, however; he took in everything with his swift, exploring eyes. His touch was light, and he moved about lightly, with a kind of lilt in his step.

Phillip, suddenly deciding he liked him, made a lunge for his knee and hung on. With this instinctive act, Phillip reassured us all that there would be no trouble or violence; Mr. Larkin would not stab anybody, or run away and hide.

Mother said that dinner would be ready in a few minutes. "Meanwhile, wouldn't you like to wash your hands, Mr. Larkin?" she asked.

"Why, no, thank you," he said.

He said it so tentatively that Mother asked him, "Are you sure?," and added, "If you should change your mind, the bathroom's through that door in the hall."

"Should I?"

"Of course not, if you don't really *want* to, Mr. Larkin."

"Maybe I should."

"All of us *always* wash our hands before going to the table," said Mother.

"Yes, certainly. Which door did you say?"

He had returned from the bathroom and was examining the piano when, without warning, Grandma Ah-Ah silently came into the parlor and so forcefully "ah-ahed" at him that he dropped the keyboard lid with a bang.

"A hundred times I've told you," she croaked.

"I'm sorry," he gasped. "I didn't know."

What Mr. Larkin didn't know was that the piano had long been her prized possession before she gave it to Mother for a wedding present, and also that this was one of her difficult days. We all knew it was, from the painful way she scowled and from the big bunch of cloth violets she wore on the top of her head.

"Grandmother, this is my friend Mr. Larkin," Father said. "He has come to have dinner with us."

"Hmm," said Grandma.

While Father said grace, I kept my head low over my plate of soup and sniffed at it. Phillip, in his high chair, banged his tray with a spoon, so that Mother had to shush him. Mr. Larkin sat across the table from Grandma Ah-Ah, very straight in her chair, as always, and her head held high. That Sunday, she gave the impression of carefully balancing the bunch of purple violets so that it would not fall off. Now and then she would hum and mumble to herself. But Mr. Larkin could not be sure it was to herself, because she stared right at him while she hummed and mumbled, and then sometimes right over his shoulder, which made him turn around to see who was there.

To take his attention from Grandma Ah-Ah, Mother told Mr. Larkin what ingredients went into her bread, and about all the things on the table that had come from her garden— tomatoes, lettuce, string beans, horseradish, currants and apples for the jellies, dill and cucumbers for the pickles. Every year, Mother dried a great deal of sweet corn, canned many other vegetables, and preserved fruits, and she listed for him all she had in her cellar, and explained her methods of canning her peas and her lima beans, preserving her strawberries, and so on.

Consuelo must have guessed from Mother's preparations that this was an unprecedented occasion and the guest an uncommon person. She wore her best fan on a long string of pink beads. Also, she had put on a perfume from Puerto Rico that made her smell like a box of Christmas chocolates. Perhaps she took an instant liking to Mr. Larkin, as Phillip had; perhaps he reminded her of her admirer in Puerto Rico; or perhaps she was bored and lonely for company there in our house in Fergus Falls. However that may be, she smiled at him invitingly again and again, rolling her eyes as she walked around the table in a new, languid manner that Mother said afterward was quite unnecessary.

After we'd had dessert, Mr. Larkin looked at his watch, then cleared his throat. He did not want to eat and run, he said, husky with shyness, but already he was expected back. He asked if he might please use the telephone to call for a livery rig.

"I'll take you in the surrey," said Father, for he was under obligation to return Mr. Larkin to the asylum himself. Though he tactfully added, "I should enjoy the drive."

"I want to go along, too," I announced.

"There is no need—" Mother began.

"Why not let him?" said Father, who seldom crossed her in family matters. "Mr. Larkin and I would like his company."

So I climbed into the back seat of the surrey, and we drove off through the Sabbath streets, past family groups sedate on open front porches, and along the shore of Lake Alice.

In his hesitating, timid way, Mr. Larkin asked Father if he was the star-gazer in the family. He said he had noted the telescope in the corner by the piano. He quoted, "Teach me your mood, O patient stars!" and asked for Father's opinion of Emerson as a poet.

Father stroked his mustache and said he read little poetry but that in the Bible. They talked of this for a while, and

"The Golden Bough," and the development of rites and beliefs in various religious faiths, which was one of Father's interests. Then inevitably Father began to speak of prophecy and divine revelation, punctuating his serene, mild speech every once in a while with an abrupt "Giddap!" and a slapping of the reins.

We were approaching the asylum grounds when Father told us two of his own experiences. As a young man, walking in the country, he had heard a Voice say "Beware!" and was saved from stepping right off a precipice; and recently, while looking ("Giddap!") through his telescope at the evening star, he had heard the same Voice, but through his own unworthiness he had failed to understand what was said.

We drove into the well-kept asylum grounds at last. Here and there, groups of lonely figures, with women nurses or men attendants in charge, were sitting, heavy and silent, on the intense-green institutional grass. Mr. Larkin turned around in the front seat to smile at me and politely ask what I wanted to be when I grew up.

"Well, I don't exactly know," I said. I scratched my head and blinked my eyes hard—two nervous mannerisms I knew were quite unnecessary. "I guess I'd like to be a trapeze acrobat," I said, blinking and scratching. "And a famous astronomer, too. But not simultaneously," I added, using a favorite word.

"Alternately," he suggested. "And correlatively."

We stopped under the great portico of the main entrance. Father told me to climb over into the front seat and hold the reins. The two men got out of the surrey and shook hands at the top of the entrance steps.

"Don't bother to come inside," Mr. Larkin told Father. "I know my way. Thank you for all your courtesy. Thank you."

He waved to me and then turned and hurried, almost ran, indoors and out of sight in the long, cool-looking corridor. And as I watched him go, I could not help but wonder if he wasn't hurrying to tell his friends about the family he had had dinner with, and act us out for their mad laughter.

PART II

Decision-making in the Community

The theme of the importance of definitional processes, begun in Part I, is continued in this section which concerns the formal decision procedures which are invoked when a person becomes known publicly as mentally ill. The first article, for purposes of contrast, describes the more informal means of handling mental illness in a small, isolated religious community. Eaton and Weil's study of the Hutterites is one of the pioneer studies of mental illness in the community, which represents a departure from the conventional clinical studies. Community studies promise to supply a new outlook on mental illness if the conceptual and methodological difficulties involved in the studies can be resolved.

The papers by Kutner and Scheff describe the operations of the courts in the screening and processing of persons who are alleged to be mentally ill. Kutner describes the procedures of the courts in Chicago, and Scheff contrasts the operations of rural and urban courts in a Midwestern state. The papers by Dinitz et al., and by Laing and Esterson describe the procedures used by the other important screening agents, the psychiatrists. Since Laing's findings are controversial, a rebuttal from the more conventional medical point of view (by Wing) is included. Although there is considerable uncertainty about some of the points discussed, all of the papers point to the central importance of community decision-making for understanding mental illness as a social problem.

The Mental Health of the Hutterites

JOSEPH W. EATON AND ROBERT J. WEIL

Is modern life driving many people insane? Would insanity diminish or disappear if mankind could return to a simpler life? From Virgil to Thoreau the philosophers have had little doubt about the answer to these questions, and some modern anthropologists have offered data which seem to bear them out. They say they have found mental disorders rare among technologically primitive peoples. For instance, recent cursory studies of the people on Okinawa and of the natives of Kenya have suggested that these groups are virtually free of some psychoses. Contrasted with this picture is the civilized United States, where some authorities have estimated that one person in 10 suffers an incapacitating mental illness at one time or another during his life.

Whether a culture can cause psychoses is not easy to discover, but one way to get at the question is to examine the mental health of a secure, stable society. The Hutterites, an isolated Anabaptist religious sect who inhabit a section of the North American Middle West, provide an ideal social laboratory of this kind. These people live a simple, rural life, have a harmonious social order and provide every member with a high level of economic security from the womb to the tomb. They are a homogeneous group, free from many of the tensions of the American melting-pot culture. And they have long been considered almost immune to mental disorders. In a study during the 1930s Lee Emerson Deets said that psychoses were almost nonexistent among them. The Manitoba Provincial Legislature received in 1947 a report which said that the Hutterites "do not contribute to the overcrowding of mental hospitals, since the mental security derived from their system results in a complete absence of mental illness."

Three years ago a research team consisting of the writers of this article—a sociologist and a psychiatrist—and the Harvard University clinical psychologists Bert Kaplan and Thomas Plant undertook a more intensive study of the Hutterites' mental health. The investigation was administered by Wayne University and financed largely by the National Institute for Mental Health. The Hutterite people cooperated generously. In the interest of science they opened their "family closets" and helped us to obtain a census of every person in their community who was then or had ever been mentally ill.

The Hutterites, whose origin as a sect goes back to 1528, are a closely knit group of German stock who had lived together in neighboring villages in Europe for a long time before they migrated to the U. S. from southern Russia between 1874 and 1877. The immigrants—101 married couples and their children—settled in eastern South Dakota. Their descendants have now spread over a wide area in the Dakotas, Montana and the prairie provinces of Canada. They live in 98 hamlets, which they call colonies. But they remain a remarkably cohesive group; each grown-up is intimately acquainted with hundreds of other members in the settlements. The Hutterites believe it sinful to marry outside the sect, and all of the present descendants (8,542 in 1950) stem from the original 101 couples.

Cardinal principles of the Hutterites are pacifism, adult baptism, the communal ownership of all property and simple living. Jewelry, art and overstuffed chairs are regarded as sinful luxuries. Radio sets and the movies are taboo. Children are the only possessions to which there is no limit: the average completed family has more than 10. The Hutterites

TABLE 1. Mental illness among United States and Canadian Hutterites living in the summer of 1951 is classified in this table. The total Hutterite population on December 31, 1950, was 8,542.

Staff Diagnosis of Illness	Lifetime Morbidity Total Number Ever Ill	Active Case Morbidity Ill in Summer 1951	Active Case Morbidity Ill but Improved on August 31, 1951	Other Cases Recovered by or before August 31, 1951	Other Cases Status Unknown
Psychoses					
Schizophrenia	9	7	1	1	0
Manic depressive reaction	39	3	5	27	4
Acute and chronic brain disorders	5	4	0	1	0
Total	53	14	6	29	4
Neuroses					
Psychoneurotic disorders	53	24	15	12	2
Psychophysiological, autonomic and visceral disorders	16	7	3	5	1
Total	69	31	18	17	3
Mental deficiency					
Mild	14	14	0	0	0
Moderate	23	23	0	0	0
Severe	14	14	0	0	0
Total	51	51	0	0	0
Epilepsy	20	12	5	3	0
Personality disorders	6	6	0	0	0
TOTAL CASES	199	114	29	49	7

cling to their own customs and are considered "different" by their neighbors. But they are not primitive in the ethnographic sense. They get a grammar-school education and speak English fluently. They read daily newspapers, have a telephone in most colonies, and own trucks. Since their own members are not encouraged to seek formal education beyond the primary grades, there are no doctors or lawyers among them, but they utilize such professional services from outside. Each hamlet engages in a highly mechanized form of agriculture. Their business with the "outside world," as Hutterites are apt to refer to their neighbors, usually exceeds $100,000 per year per colony.

On the surface it seemed that the Hutterites did indeed enjoy extraordinary freedom from mental illness. We did not find a single Hutterite in a mental hospital. The 55 outside doctors patronized by these people said they showed fewer psychosomatic and nervous symptoms than their neighbors of other faiths. But this appearance of unusual mental health did not stand the test of an intensive screening of the inhabitants, carried out colony by colony. Among the 8,542 Hutterites we discovered a total of 199 (1 in 43) who either had active symptoms of a mental disorder or had recovered from such an illness. Of these illnesses 53 were diagnosed as psychoses, all but five of them of a functional (non-organic) character.

In short, the Hutterite culture provides no immunity to mental disorders. The existence of these illnesses in so secure and stable a social order suggests that there may be genetic, organic, or constitutional predispositions to psychosis which will cause breakdowns among individuals in any society, no matter how protective and well integrated.

The distribution of symptoms among the Hutterites was quite unusual. There were few cases diagnosed as schizophrenia, although elsewhere this is the most common psychosis. Only nine Hutterites had ever manifested the pattern of delusions, hallucinations and other recognized symptoms of schizophrenia; the group lifetime rate was 2.1 per 1,000 persons aged 15 and over. On the other hand, the proportion of manic-depressive reactions among those with mental disorders was unusual; this disorder accounted for

39 of the 53 psychoses, and the rate was 9.3 per 1,000 aged 15 and over. The name of the disorder is misleading; manic-depressives often are not dangerous to other persons, and none of the Hutterite patients was. Their symptoms were predominantly depressive. There was much evidence of irrational guilt feelings, self-blame, withdrawal from normal social relations and marked slowing of mental and motor activities. Five of the patients had suicidal impulses. Two Hutterites had actually killed themselves.

The fact that in the Hutterite society manic-depression is more common than schizophrenia, reversing the situation in all other populations for whom comparable data have been obtained, suggests that cultural factors do have some influence on the manifestation of psychoses. A Johns Hopkins University team of researchers who recently made an extensive analysis of mental hospital statistics concluded that schizophrenic symptoms are most common among unskilled laborers, farmers, urban residents in rooming-house sections and other persons who are relatively isolated socially, while manic-depressive reactions are more prevalent among professional, socially prominent, and religious persons, who have a stronger need to live up to social expectations. Our data fit this theory well. Religion is the focus of the Hutterite way of life. Their whole educational system, beginning with nursery school, orients the people to look for blame and guilt within themselves rather than in others. Physical aggression is taboo. Like the Catholic orders, Hutterites own everything in the name of their church. They eat in a common dining room, pay medical bills from the communal treasury and work at jobs assigned to them by managers elected by the males of the colony. The group, rather than the individual, comes first.

In projective psychological tests the Hutterites, like other groups, show anti-social and aggressive impulses, but in their daily lives they repress these effectively. Their history showed no case of murder, arson, severe physical assault or sex crime. No individual warranted the diagnosis of psychopath. Divorce, desertion, separation or chronic marital discord were rare. Only five marriages were known to have gone on the rocks since 1875. Personal violence and childish or amoral forms of behavior among adults were uncommon, even in persons with psychotic episodes. There were no psychoses stemming from drug addiction, alcoholism, or syphilis, although these disorders account for approximately 10 percent of all first admissions to state mental hospitals in the United States. In general our study tends to confirm the theory of many social scientists and public health officials that a favorable cultural setting can largely prevent these forms of social maladjustment.

All this does not entirely rule out the possibility that genetic factors play some part in the unusual proportions of manic-depression and schizophrenia symptoms among the Hutterites. There is some evidence that these disorders tend to run in families. The Hutterites are biologically inbred. Three surnames—Hofer, Waldner and Wipt—accounted for nearly half of all families in 1950. It is possible that the Hutterite group has a disproportionate number of persons genetically prone to becoming depressed—if there is such a predisposition. A team of Harvard University workers is planning to make a follow-up genetic study of the Hutterites.

The question of the relation of mental disorders to culture is difficult to investigate quantitatively. No country has a really complete record of mental disorders among its population. Censuses of patients in mental hospitals are almost worthless for this purpose; they leave out patients who have recovered and mentally ill persons who have never come to the attention of doctors.

The Hutterite study attempted to track down every case of a mental disorder, past or present, hospitalized or not, in the whole living population. It probably succeeded in finding virtually all the cases of psychosis. Similar studies have been made of seven other communities in various parts of the world, and the results are shown in the tables on page 101. They give the comparative rates of psychosis, as standardized by the Hutterite lifetime rate and corrected for variations in age and sex distribution. (The Hutterite population is predominantly youthful—50 percent under 15 years of age.)

On this basis the Hutterites apparently rank second highest among the eight populations in the rate of psychosis, being exceeded only by an area in the north of Sweden. But there is considerable evidence that the count of mental disorders was less complete in the other seven groups; that is, in those studies many cases were missed because their illness was not a matter of public record, while the Hutterite population was thoroughly screened. It is probable that the psychosis rate among the Hutterites is actually low compared with that in other populations. It seems to be only one third as high as the rate in New York State, for instance, taking into consideration the common estimate that even in that State (where mental hospital facilities are among the most extensive) there is at least one undetected psychotic person for every one in an institution.

The statistical comparison of mental disorder rates has many limitations, but it does offer several promising leads to the puzzle that the problem of functional psychoses presents to modern science. Among the Hutterites, as in all the other populations, the frequency of psychoses increases rapidly with age. Among those who showed manic-depressive reactions, females predominated. The social biology of the aging process and of sex probably holds worthwhile clues to some of the problems of cause and treatment.

Neuroses were more common than psychoses among the Hutterites, as elsewhere. Four fifths of the 69 discovered neurotics were female. Melancholy moods were regarded by teachers as the number one emotional problem of Hutterite school children. Hutterite neurotics showed the same tendency as psychotics to take out mental stress on themselves instead of on others. Self-blame and remorse were common, as were psychosomatic headaches, backaches and hysteric paralysis of a limb. There was little scapegoating or projection of hostile feelings by imputing them to others.

There is no evidence of any unusual concentration of hereditary mental defects in the Hutterite population. A total of 51 persons was diagnosed as mentally deficient, and 20 normal persons had suffered epileptic attacks. These epilepsy and mental deficiency rates are not high in comparison with other groups.

How does the Hutterite culture deal with mental illness? Although it does not prevent mental disorders, it provides a highly therapeutic atmosphere for their treatment. The onset of a symptom serves as a signal to the entire community to demonstrate support and love for the patient. Hutterites do not approve of the removal of any member to a "strange" hospital, except for short periods to try shock treatments. All patients are looked after by the immediate family. They are treated as ill rather than "crazy." They are encouraged to participate in the normal life of their family and community, and most are able to do some useful work. Most of the manic-depressive patients get well, but among neurotic patients recovery is less common. Most of the epileptics were either cured or took drugs which greatly relieved the condition. No permanent stigma is attached to patients after recovery. The traumatic social consequences which a mental disorder usually brings to the patient, his family and sometimes his community are kept to a minimum by the patience and tolerance with which most Hutterites regard these conditions. This finding supports the theory that at least some of the severely antisocial forms of behavior usually displayed by psychotic and disturbed patients are not an inherent attribute. They may be reflections of the impersonal manner of handling patients in most mental hospitals, of their emotional rejection by the family and of their stigmatization in the community.

In the Hutterite social order people are exposed to a large number of common experiences. Their indoctrination begins in infancy and is continued by daily religious instruction and later by daily church-going. Hutterites spend their entire life within a small and stable group. Their homes consist only of bedrooms, all furnished in an almost identical manner. The women take turns cooking and baking for everybody. Everyone wears the same kind of clothes; the women, for example, all let their hair grow without cutting, part it in the middle and cover it with a black kerchief with white polka dots. The Hutterite religion provides definite answers for many of the problems that come up.

Despite this uniformity in the externals of living, Hutterites are not stereotyped personalities. Differences in genetic, organic and psychological factors seem to be sufficiently powerful to produce an infinite variety of behavior, even in a social order as rigid as this one. It appears that the nightmare of uniformity sketched in George Orwell's *Nineteen Eighty-four* is actually unachievable in a living society. At least our study in depth disclosed no simple standardization of personality structure among Hutterites.

There is considerable objective evidence that the great majority of Hutterites have a high level of psychological adjustment. Their misfortunes and accidents are alleviated greatly by the group's system of mutual aid. The sick, the aged, the widows and orphans are well taken care of. In the last three decades only about 100 persons (most of them male) have left the community permanently. During World War II about one third of the men between the ages of 20 and 40 served in camps for conscientious objectors; more than 98 percent of them ultimately returned to their colonies.

There has not, however, been any rush of applicants from outside to join the Hutterite sect. Mental health involves value judgments and depends on what people want from life. Only 19 adults have joined the sect in America during the last few decades. The austere and puritanical customs of the sect impose restrictions which even the members, who learn to accept them, regard as a "narrow path." Their culture is therapeutic only for conformists. There are occasional rebels; the more able ones find a means of expressing themselves by becoming leaders, the less brilliant have difficulties.

The survival of this 16th-century peasant culture in the heart of the most 20th-century-minded continent is a vivid demonstration of the power of values and beliefs. Although our data on the Hutterites' mental disorders clearly demonstrate the inadequacy of a purely cultural approach to the problem of mental health, they do show that culture has a large influence in shaping personality. Psychiatrists who work exclusively in hospitals or clinics cannot see the whole patient as he functions in his total environment. Our findings lead us to conclude that the social relations of the patient and his culture, including the things in which he believes, deserve more attention from psychiatric researchers and clinicians than is commonly given to them.

TABLE 2. Eight groups investigated by independent studies, including the one described here, are analyzed for percentage of each major diagnostic category among their psychotics.

| Study | Number of Cases Diagnosed | Percent of Cases Diagnosed | | | |
		Schizo-phrenia	Manic Depression	All Other Diagnoses	TOTAL
Ethnic Hutterites	53	17	74	9	100
North Swedish Area	107	87	2	11	100
West Swedish Island of Abo	94	43	27	30	100
Bornholm Island	481	31	25	43	100
Williamson County, Tenn.	156	27	26	47	100
Baltimore Eastern Health District	367	43	11	46	100
Thuringian Villages	200	37	10	53	100
Bavarian Villages, Rosenheim Area	21	38	10	52	100

TABLE 3. One group, the Hutterites, is compared to the other seven by the standard expectancy method. The frequency of *diagnosed* cases of psychosis among Hutterites is relatively high.

Survey	Total Population	Actual Number of Cases Found	Expected Number of Cases by Hutterites Norms	Expectancy Ratio
North Swedish Area	8,651	107	94	1.14
Ethnic Hutterites	8,542	53	53	1.00
Bornholm Island	45,694	481	773	.62
Baltimore Eastern Health District	55,129	507	822	.62
Williamson County, Tenn.	24,804	156	271	.58
West Swedish Island of Abo	8,735	94	186	.51
Bavarian Villages, Rosenheim Area	3,203	21	49	.43
Thuringian Villages	37,546	200	617	.32

The Illusion of Due Process in Commitment Proceedings

LUIS KUTNER

> Psychology has as much to
> gain from studying the opera-
> tion of law as law has to gain
> from greater appreciation of
> psychology.
>
> **DAVID RIESMAN**

INTRODUCTION

Procedures in the United States for committing the mentally ill are sick, obsolescent, and unjust. Conceived in an era when the diagnosis and treatment of mental illness were little understood, and since then subjected to countless alterations, amendments, and revisions, the commitment procedures of most states stand today as mighty monuments of complexity, yet remain inadequate in both medical and legal eyes. Indeed, elaborate statutory provisions for the protection of the individual are often mere illusions of due process, as many pressures, particularly the demands of medical propriety, require that "legalistic" corners be cut. The cause of

FROM *Northwestern University Law Review* 57 (September–October, 1962) 383–99. The section reprinted here is the first 6 pages of the above article. Reprinted by permission of the author and the publisher. Some footnotes are omitted. Assistance of Russell M. Pelton, University of Chicago School of Law, and Charlotte Ziporyn, LL.B., is acknowledged.

this confusion is the complete lack of understanding between the medical and legal professions with regard to commitment of the mentally ill. It is the purpose of this article to point out some of the conflicts and contradictions within the commitment procedure, and perhaps, in a small way, to contribute to mutual understanding and respect between medicine and the law, with a resultant improvement in the application of due process by the commitment machinery.

On October 5, 1960, Mrs. Anna Duzynski, a recent Polish emigrant who lived with her husband on the northwest side of Chicago, discovered that $380 in cash had been stolen from her apartment. Suspecting that the money had been taken by the building janitor, the only other person who had a key to the apartment, Mrs. Duzynski rushed to his flat and demanded that the money be returned. The janitor in turn called the police, and upon their arrival stated that both Mr. and Mrs. Duzynski were insane and should be committed to a mental institution. Without any further examination, the police seized both Anna and Michael Duzynski, neither of whom spoke English, and took them in handcuffs to the Cook County Mental Health Clinic. At the Mental Health Clinic, unable to answer questions in English and thereby defend themselves, the Duzynskis were duly pronounced mentally ill and committed to the Chicago State Hospital. Six weeks later, Michael Duzynski still had less idea why he had been imprisoned than he had when thrown into a Nazi concentration camp in World War II. Finally, in desperation, he hanged himself. The gross injustice of the entire affair thus vividly pointed out to them, hospital officials hurriedly released Anna Duzynski the next day.[1]

The significance of this case lies not only in the fact that it demonstrates that people are still trying to "railroad" others into mental institutions, but also in the fact that in a supposedly enlightened state such as Illinois[2] this "railroading" attempt was successful. The woman involved owes her present liberty not to any procedural "safeguards" in the Illinois Mental Health Code, but rather to her husband's tragic death which pointed out the injustice of their confinement. Thus, more than anything else, the Duzynski case illustrates a great weakness in the commitment procedure of Illinois as well as that of most other states; i.e., a great discrepancy between the theoretical (statutory) and the practical ways in which persons are committed to mental institutions. The legal profession laboriously constructs elaborate provisions to guarantee that no person shall be committed without "due process of law"; then the medical profession quietly circumvents much of this procedural "red tape" because of the requirements of medical propriety. The result is often that while numerous statutory provisions can be cited which apparently guarantee protection of the individual's liberty, in actual practice such statutes are mere illusions of due process.

ILLINOIS TYPIFIES THE ILLUSION OF DUE PROCESS

Illinois is a classic example of a state in which there is great variance between the statutory and the actual commitment procedures. The Illinois Mental Health Code provides a series of safeguards which seem to insure that no sane person will ever be committed to an institution for the mentally ill. Before any person can be involuntarily committed to a state institution, the code requires: (a) a petition signed by a friend or relative of the alleged-mentally-ill, stating that the petitioner knows the person threatened with confinement and believes him to be mentally ill, (b) a physician's certificate stating that the "patient" is mentally ill; (c) an examination by one or more court-appointed doctors, who will prepare a diagnosis and submit it to the court; and (d) a court hearing at which the alleged-mentally-ill is entitled to demand a jury. While this system appears on paper to fully protect the rights of the sane, in actual practice many pressures, particularly the demands of medical propriety, reduce the procedural safeguards to meaningless gestures.

The sharp dichotomy between the statutory and actual commitment procedures in Illinois is best illustrated by the following examples of the Cook County Mental Health Clinic in operation.[3] (1) To satisfy the "formality" of a physician's certification of insanity, the certificates are signed as a matter of course by staff physicians of the Mental Health Clinic after little or no examination and after the alleged-mentally-ill has *already* been brought in for confinement. Moreover, the *same* staff doctor is one of those later appointed to handle the examination for the court,[4] eliminating the possibility of one doctor acting as a check upon another, which is the very purpose of requiring *two* medical examinations. (2) As might be expected, the examination by the state physicians is given great, if not decisive, weight at the court hearing. The flaw is that the so-called "examinations" are made on an assembly-line basis, *often being completed in two or three minutes, and never taking more than ten minutes.* Although psychiatrists agree that it is practically impossible to determine a person's sanity on the basis of such a short and hurried interview, doctors at the Mental Health Clinic recommend confinement in 77% of the cases.[5] It appears that in practice the alleged-mentally-ill is presumed to be insane and bears the burden of proving his sanity in the few minutes allotted him. (3) A person's last opportunity to demonstrate his sanity is at the court hearing, yet doctors at the Mental Health Clinic keep all the "patients" under such heavy sedation that many of them appear stuporous at their hearings and are unable to intelligently defend themselves for that reason alone.[6] (4) It is apparently the practice of the Clinic not to notify persons threatened with incarceration of their right to counsel or a jury trial, and indeed to reprimand or dismiss workers who do inform the alleged-mentally-ill of their legal rights.[7]

Viewed in this light, the elaborate due process provisions of the Illinois Mental Health Code become a mockery. Nor is this problem native to Illinois alone, as a study of the case law indicates its presence in numerous American jurisdictions.[8] The cause of this lack of conformity between the law and its application is the simple fact that confinement of the mentally ill has long been a battleground between the medical and legal professions. Each side has insisted on the legislative acceptance of its basic tenets, while ignoring equally valid points raised by the other side. The medical profession insists that the law remain as informal and flexible as possible, arguing that excessive legal formality is harmful to the welfare of the "patient." The legal profession, on the other hand, insists that a fair hearing on notice, the right to counsel, and the right to a jury trial are fundamental principles of justice which our law guarantees to all persons threatened with incarceration, including those faced with involuntary confinement in mental institutions.[9] This conflict of philosophies has not only led to confusion in the formation and execution of mental health programs, but it is also the prime reason for the present failure of commitment practices to conform with the statutory requirements for commitment.

THE MEDICAL–LEGAL CONFLICT

For years legal scholars have insisted that persons threatened with confinement in mental institutions be given the same procedural safeguards as persons threatened with criminal incarceration. The law is not yet convinced that, even under modern practices, commitment to a mental institution is more analogous to hospitalization than it is to criminal imprisonment. Indeed, the degree of confinement, the loss of civil rights, the inability of the confined to communicate easily with the outside, and the resulting social ostracism, all tend to support the law's insistence that involuntary commitment to a mental institution is by its very nature quite analogous to imprisonment. The position of the legal profession has perhaps best been summarized by Weihofen and Overholser, as follows:

Despite the impatience of medical men and others with legal practices, it is nevertheless true that legal "technicalities" represent the lawmakers' effort to apply principles of fairness and justice in dealing with human rights which have been established only by the blood and sweat of bygone generations who saw and suffered the effects of more summary methods. It is a precious heritage that gives us the right to insist that a man be served with notice of the pendency of any legal action in which his rights may be affected, and have opportunity to be present, confront and cross-examine those who give testimony against him, and introduce any testimony he may have in his own defense— instead of having his rights decided in a secret "star chamber" proceeding, and his life or liberty taken from him by a *lettre de cachet* calling for his confinement or liquidation without notice or hearing. The terms "star chamber" and *lettre de cachet* describe no imaginary evils dreamed up by cautious lawyers, but very real practices current not so many hundreds of years ago, and hardly exceeded in arbitrariness, tyranny and injustice by practices rampant in Germany and elsewhere in our own times.

Safeguards designed to guarantee fair procedure and to prevent the abuse of commitments laws . . . are therefore not mere technicalities and formalities to be lightly pushed aside in favor of some summary commitment procedure.

The great fear of the legal profession, of course, is that without adequate procedural safeguards perfectly sane members of society may be "railroaded" into mental institutions by unscrupulous relatives or business associates. An example of such a situation was the Illinois case of *Brandt* v. *Brandt,* in which a husband, having an affair with another woman, arranged to have his wife committed to a mental institution. Although proven cases of "railroading" are rather rare, the legal profession believes that enough cases of either intentional or negligent confinement of sane persons have been recorded to warrant the retention of procedural safeguards in this area.

On the other hand, the medical profession is quite right in maintaining that excessive legal formality may do positive harm to the mental patient. A former president of the American Psychiatric Association pointed out the defects in the ordinary forms of judicial procedure when applied to the determination of mental illness thus:

Not long ago in California a wife decided that her husband was mentally sick. He was depressed and had delusions that persons were trying to kill him. Following the regular legal procedure, she swore out a warrant, the sheriff arrested the patient, and he was taken to the county jail, there to await a hearing before the judge. That night he hanged himself in the jail. To those sticklers for legal procedure and defense of the legal rights of the patient, I would point out that his legal rights were well preserved. He was arrested on a warrant by a sheriff; he was not sent to a hospital without due process of law and a chance to appear before the judge. Perhaps if he had, he might be alive today. The point I wish to make is that the public is so obsessed with the legal point of view and the alleged infallibility of legal procedure that they insist on protecting the so-called legal rights of the patient without thinking of what his medical rights are.

Lost in the swirl of argument between the two disciplines is the simple fact that confinement of the mentally ill is not exclusively a legal or a medical problem, but is in fact a combination of both. The amorphous relationship here between medicine and the law has perhaps best been stated as follows:

Mental illness, as such, like any other illness, is a medical problem and is primarily of concern to the medical profession. . . . One of the principal characteristics of mental illness, or possibly even a definition, is the failure of the individual to adapt to the society of which he is a part. Whether the illness results from organic causes, such as paresis, or is one of the diseases for which no organic cause can be found, the symptoms of serious mental illness are essentially those of release, or regression to an uninhibited state. The social controls, including the individual's ability to work within a complex human relationship, are usually the first to suffer deterioration. This failure may result in the inability of the individual to care for himself, or it may be expressed in antisocial conduct directed at others. In either case, the problems are no longer medical, but have social and legal consequences. Thus the law, which is the most specialized and coercive of social controls is used to regulate and channel the by-products of mental illness.[10]

Thus, recognizing the validity of the basic positions of both the medical and legal professions, the problem is twofold: First, to restrain the law from constructing commitment procedures which are medically unreasonable; and second, to convince the medical profession that it must fully comply with commitment procedures which are enacted. The key to the solution of these problems is simply that both disciplines must be made to appreciate the inherent equity and logic in the other's position.

. . .

Social Conditions for Rationality:
How Urban and Rural Courts
Deal with the Mentally Ill

THOMAS J. SCHEFF

Formal legal procedure is a highly developed instrument for arriving at rational decisions concerning complex and uncertain situations. Legal procedures are institutionalized means for substantial rationality, i.e., for obtaining "intelligent insight into the inter-relations of events in a given situation."[1] Like scientific method, trial procedures and due process serve to control and reduce, though not to eliminate, bias in situations of uncertainty.

One of the central concerns in the sociology of knowledge has been the attempt to determine the social conditions under which substantial rationality occurs. This paper pursues the question by discussing some of the variation in the procedures for hospitalizing and committing persons alleged to be mentally ill, in metropolitan and non-metropolitan jurisdictions in a Midwestern state. My sources of information were interviews with judges, psychiatrists, and other officials in 20 of its counties and observations of judicial hearings, psychiatric interviews, and other procedures in four of the jurisdictions, those courts with the largest number of mental hearings.[2]

From the *American Behavioral Scientist* 7 (March, 1964) 21–27. Reprinted by permission of the author and the publisher.

NON-RATIONAL PROCEDURES AND
URBAN COURTS

The major result of our study was the conclusion that in three of the four metropolitan courts, the civil procedures for hospitalizing and committing the mentally ill had no serious investigatory purpose, but were ceremonial in character. Although all four of the courts carried through various procedures required by statute, the psychiatric examination, the judicial hearing, and other steps, hospitalization and treatment appeared to be virtually automatic after the patient had been brought to the attention of the courts.[3]

In nine of the 16 other counties, however, these civil procedures appeared to serve at least some investigatory purpose. At one or more points in the screening process (the application for judicial inquiry, the psychiatric examination, the judicial hearing) detailed investigation was conducted and patients were released or their release was seriously considered.

These observations suggest that for civil procedures concerning mental illness, rationality is associated with a non-metropolitan setting, and bias and the presumption of illness with metropolitan jurisdictions. Before exploring some of the reasons for this relationship, it is necessary to justify the contention that the procedures used in the metropolitan jurisdictions are not rational.

Most of the officials whom we interviewed did not disagree with our description of the typical events in these procedures, but argued that the procedures were justified by larger considerations of a medical and humanitarian character. Their arguments can be summarized in the following five statements:

1. The condition of mentally ill persons deteriorates rapidly without psychiatric assistance.
2. Effective psychiatric treatments exist for most mental illnesses.
3. Unlike surgery, there are no risks involved in involuntary psychiatric treatment: it either helps or is neutral, it can't hurt.
4. Exposing a prospective mental patient to questioning, cross-examination, and other screening procedures exposes him to the unneces-

sary stigma of trial-like procedures, and may do further damage to his mental condition.

5. There is an element of danger to self or others in mental illness. It is better to risk unnecessary hospitalization than the harm the patient might do himself or others.

Although these statements appear to be plausible, statements rebutting each of them are equally plausible.

1. The assumption that psychiatric disorders usually get worse without treatment rests on very little other than evidence of an anecdotal character. There is just as much evidence that most acute psychological and emotional upsets are self-terminating.[4]
2. It is still not clear, according to systematic studies evaluating psychotherapy, drugs, etc., that most psychiatric interventions are any more effective, on the average, than no treatment at all.[5]
3. There is very good evidence that involuntary hospitalization may affect the patient's life—his job, his family affairs, etc. There is some evidence that too hasty exposure to psychiatric treatment may convince the patient that he is "sick," prolonging what might have been an otherwise transitory episode.[6]
4. This assumption is correct, as far as it goes. But it is misleading because it fails to consider what occurs when the patient who does not wish to be hospitalized is forcibly treated. Such patients often become extremely indignant and angry, particularly in the event, which is common, that they are deceived into coming to the hospital on a pretext.
5. The element of danger is usually exaggerated both in amount and degree. In the psychiatric survey of new patients in state mental hospitals, conducted as part of the present study, danger to self or others was mentioned in less than a fourth of the cases. Furthermore, in those cases where danger is mentioned, it is not always clear that the risks involved are greater than those encountered in ordinary social life. This issue has been discussed by Ross, an attorney: A truck driver with a mild neurosis who is "accident prone" is probably a greater danger to society than most psychotics; yet, he will not be committed for treatment, even if he would be benefited. The community expects a certain amount of dangerous activity. I suspect that as a class, drinking drivers are a greater danger than the mentally ill, and yet the drivers are tolerated or punished with small fines rather than indeterminate imprisonment.[7]

These latter five statements indicate that arriving at a rational decision concerning hospitalization is not usually a simple and expedient matter. In marginal cases, which frequently arise, a rational disposition would require careful investigation and assessment. Yet in many of the marginal cases we observed, investigation and assessment were quite limited or absent entirely. Some examples of the attitudes and actions of the officials illustrate this point.

EXAMINATION AND HEARING

The examination by the psychiatrists in the urban courts virtually never led to extensive knowledge of the facts. These examinations appeared to be short (about 10 minutes on the average), hurried, and largely routine. Yet the psychiatrists we interviewed uniformly stated that such a short interview was almost worthless with all but the most extreme cases.

One of the examiners, after stating in an interview (before we observed his examinations) that he usually took about thirty minutes, stated: "It's not remunerative. I'm taking a hell of a cut. I can't spend 45 minutes with a patient. I don't have the time, it doesn't pay." In the examinations that we observed, this physician actually spent 8, 10, 5, 8, 8, 7, 17, and 11 minutes with the patients, or an average of 9.2 minutes.

The key step in the entire sequence is the judicial hearing. Yet these hearings were usually limited to the minimum act required by statute. In one urban court (the court with the largest number of cases) the only contact between the judge and the patient was in a preliminary hearing. This hearing was held with such lightning rapidity (1.6 minutes average) and followed such a standard and unvarying format that it was obvious that the judge made no attempt to use the hearing results in arriving at a decision. He asked three questions uniformly: "How are you feeling?" "How are you being treated?", and "If the doctors recommend that you stay here a while, would you cooperate?" No matter how the patient responded, the judge immediately signified that the hearing was over, cutting off some of the patients in the middle of a sentence.

Even in those courts where some attempt was made to ascertain the circumstances surrounding the case, the judge did not appear to assess the meaning of the circumstances in order to make a rational disposition. For example, in another urban court, the judge seemed to use the hearing to gather information. He attempted to relax the patient, reassure him, get his point of view, and test his orientation. (Of the four courts, the hearings in this court lasted longest: 12 minutes average, as against 1.6, 6, and 9 minutes in the other three courts.) Yet in all the hearings we observed (43), including those in which the judge himself demonstrated that the patient's behavior and orientation were unexceptionable, the judge went on to commit to or continue hospitalization.

The way in which this same judge reacted to a difficult case can be used to illustrate another facet of the concept of substantial rationality. The examining psychiatrists had recommended commitment for the patient, a policeman, whom they had diagnosed as severely depressed. Another psychiatrist (not one of the examiners) had once told the judge that there was always the risk of suicide in severe depression. This patient, however, had no history of suicide attempts, and strenuously denied any suicidal intention. The patient had retained his own attorney (which is unusual) who pleaded at the hearing that the patient be released to the care of a private physician, because if he were commited he would almost certainly lose his job. The judge refused to consider the plea stating that if there were *any* risk of suicide, he did not want to be responsible for having released the patient.

Reaching a decision in this case could never be a simple matter, since it requires the evaluation and comparison of a number of disparate considerations: what is the likelihood that the patient would commit suicide if released? Is this likelihood greater than those which are or should be tolerated in the community? What is the likelihood that the patient would lose his job if committed? How should this likelihood be weighed relative to the likelihood of suicide? This latter question particularly is a complex question, involving joint consideration of likelihoods and "costs" of seemingly incommensurate events. Decisions which meet the criteria of substantial rationality thus require consideration of diverse kinds of information, and equally important, the judicious comparison and weighing of the information.

THE ATTEMPT AT RATIONALITY
IN RURAL COURTS

In some of the non-metropolitan counties we investigated, these kinds of questions were addressed to some degree. In the application for judicial inquiry or in the judicial hearing, or, in two jurisdictions, in the psychiatric screening, serious investigation and assessment were undertaken. In three of the less populated counties, the judge himself heard the testimony before the application for judicial inquiry, and in some cases had the county sheriff or other officer investigate the situation even before issuing an application. In the hearing, several of the judges required that the relatives and the examining psychiatrists be present, allowing for the possibility of confrontation and cross-examination.

It is also true, however, that the procedures in three of the non-metropolitan counties were even more peremptory than in the metropolitan courts. In these three courts, the person alleged to be mentally ill was simply conveyed to the distant state mental hospital, after the application for judicial inquiry had been accepted, without examination or hearing. This occurred even though the Attorney General had issued the opinion that this procedure was illegal.

Allowing for a number of such exceptions, the findings discussed above point to the absence of substantial rationality in the metropolitan courts, and the presence of a degree of rationality in the non-metropolitan courts. On the basis of this relationship, we can now consider some of the conditions which facilitate and impede substantial rationality.

CONDITIONS FAVORING SUBSTANTIAL
RATIONALITY

Although we ordinarily think of the metropolitan court as being richer in resources than the rural court, there is one commodity which is very rare in the city, *time*. The metropolitan courts are faced with an enormous volume of cases: court B, the extreme example, handled some 14,000 cases (mostly misdemeanors) in 1962. In these circumstances, and with limited numbers of court officers, individual attention to a single case is usually not feasible.

The second condition concerns political pressure. In both rural and metropolitan courts there is considerable public sentiment about cases in which the judge or other official errs by releasing a person whom subsequent events prove should have been retained. There is considerably less sentiment against the opposite error, of retaining a person who should have been released. Officials therefore appear much more careful about erroneously releasing than they are about erroneously retaining. Our impression, however, was that this is less of an issue in rural areas. The absence of sensational treatment of mistakes in the newspapers, and the generally greater personal familiarity with facts of the case, makes for less political pressure on the rural judge.

Court officials in rural areas also usually have greater personal familiarity with the situation than do urban judges. In the typical rural case the judge will personally know the person alleged to be mentally ill, or at least a member of his family. This greater familiarity may lead to delay and investigation that would be absent in the urban court, where virtually every person who comes before the court is a stranger.

Personal familiarity with the patient affects not only the official's knowledge about the patient, but also his attitude. From our interviews, we gained the impression that it was much easier for the officials to consider cases using the impersonal framework of mental illness if they did not know the patient personally. This consideration operated in conjunction with the fact that the rural judges tended to be less psychiatrically sophisticated than the judges in the metropolitan courts, and to use a commonsense framework in most cases.

A fourth condition is also related to the ideological framework within which the officials considered the case. The greater psychiatric sophistication of the metropolitan judges reduces the rationality of their decision procedures in two ways. By establishing the assumption that the person alleged to be mentally ill is "sick" and in "need of help," extra-legal humanitarian considerations are introduced, and tend to break down the investigatory and adjudicatory nature of the court procedures. Introduction of the idea of disease also diffuses the responsibility for a final decision between the judge, who has the legal authority for the decision, and the psychiatrist, whom the judge assumes to have authority by virtue of his technical knowledge. We received the impression that the consequence of this diffusion of authority is that neither the judge nor the psychiatrist assumes the responsibility for decision to continue hospitalization, but each believes that his own decision is unimportant, since the real authority rests with the other.

A final condition is related to the resources of the patient. We formed the impression that an articulate patient, who knew his rights and who had the ability to retain his own lawyer, had a much better chance to obtain summary release from the hospital than the patient who was inarticulate, was unaware of his legal rights, and did not have the money or knowledge to retain a lawyer to represent him.

THE INCIDENCE OF MENTAL ILLNESS

To summarize these five conditions, we found that in jurisdictions characterized by a small volume of cases, only moderate public pressures against releasing patients erroneously, personal acquaintance with the patient or his family, little psychiatric sophistication, and where the patient has resources for defending himself against the allegations about him, substantial rationality is a characteristic of civil commitment procedures. In jurisdictions with large numbers of cases, strong public pressures against erroneous releases, lack of personal acquaintance with the persons alleged to be mentally ill, and few resources for patients to defend themselves against the allegations, hospitalization and treatment are virtually automatic once the complaint has been made to the court.

To the extent that all five of the latter conditions are present, hospitalization, far from being a rational decision, becomes an irreversible process. Since the procedures used in the metropolitan areas account for the majority of patients coming to the mental hospitals, the irreversibility of hospitalization has implications which deserve more attention than can be given them here. First, this discussion suggests that the well-established relationship between urban areas and high rates of mental illness may be a product less of greater incidence of mental illness than of the absence of official screening in urban areas.

Secondly, and more generally, since the entire legal and medical decision-making process in metropolitan areas appears to be largely ceremonial, the important decision in hospitalization is that which is made before the complaint comes to the court, i.e., in the community, and particularly in the family. The crucial decision of diagnosis, hospitalization, and treatment is thus made usually not by an expert, but by a layman: the relatives or others who bring the case before the court. This suggests that understanding of the incidence of mental illness requires study of the operation of social control in the community.

CONDITIONS FOR RATIONALITY
IN OTHER SETTINGS

Turning from the topic of decision-making in mental illness to broader concerns, it might be worthwhile to consider some of the conditions discussed here in connection with rationality in other areas. The recent New York bail studies suggest that much of the same situation applies to the handling of criminal deviants in the New York legal system as was discussed here.[8] Decisions concerning scientific matters may also be usefully considered within this framework. The decisions of an advisory board evaluating research findings, or, more frequently, research proposals, might be analysed in this way, to ascertain the effect of volume of cases, political pressure because of erroneous decisions, the ideological framework of the members of the board, the diffusion of responsibility, the effect of personal acquaintance with the applicants, and the power and resources available to the applicants.

A pair of examples will illustrate one of the many parallels between judicial and scientific decision-making which bear on the issue of the conditions for rationality. The diffusion of responsibility between the judge and the psychiatrist, discussed above, puts the judge in the position of having the legal, but not the technical, authority to make final dispositions in hospitalization and commitment. Apparently, however, this conflict is consciously used by some judges who privately have doubts about the seriousness of the psychiatric examination. These judges justify their decisions by referring to the recommendations of the psychiatrists, and thus use the psychiatrists as "fronts" for their own purposes.

Apparently, like psychiatry, the name of science is regularly invoked as a bureaucratic mechanism of defense. The following testimony is by a missile expert, Werner von Braun, before a congressional investigating committee:[9]

> . . . a physics professor may know a lot about the upper atmosphere, but when it comes to making a sound appraisal of what missile schedule is sound and how you can phase a research and development program into industrial production, he is pretty much at a loss. . . . When confronted with a difficult decision involving several hundred million dollars, and of vital importance to the national defense, many Pentagon executives like to protect themselves. It helps if a man can say, "I have on my advisory committee some Nobel prize winners, or some very famous people that everybody knows." And if these famous people then sign a final recommendation, the executive feels, "Now, if something goes wrong, nobody can blame me for not having asked the smartest men in the country what they think about this."

The parallel suggested by these two examples points to regularized organizational techniques for manipulating avowedly rational means to serve non-rational ends, and suggests the need for studies explicitly formulated to determine the social conditions for substantial rationality. Although rationality is a difficult and elusive concept, such studies could help to clarify it and bring empirical materials to bear on an important problem.

Psychiatric and Social Attributes as Predictors of Case Outcome in Mental Hospitalization

*SIMON DINITZ, MARK LEFTON, SHIRLEY
ANGRIST AND BENJAMIN PASAMANICK*

A continuing source of difficulty in mental health research, as in many other aspects of the behavioral sciences, is the chronic inability to predict behavior prospectively. The difficulty in accurately predicting case outcome is particularly acute in the institutional area where an ever increasing number of persons must be cared for and treated and where decisions must constantly be made about readiness for discharge based upon reasonably efficient criteria of outcome.

The difficulty in predicting post-hospital adjustment derives in part from the lack of understanding of the etiology of most of the mental diseases. It also derives to a considerable extent, however, from the variety and diversity of objective and subjective factors—prehospital, hospital and posthospital—which seem to play some role, singly and in combination, in determining posthospital success and failure and adequacy of functioning.

These formidable obstacles, fortunately, have not pre-

FROM *Social Problems* 8 (Spring, 1961) 322–328. Reprinted by permission of the author and the publisher.

The outcome study reported in this paper was made possible by a National Institute of Mental Health grant, M-2953. During the course of the study, S. Angrist held a pre-doctoral fellowship from NIMH, United States Public Health Service.

vented researchers from investigating prehospital, and post-hospital variables as they may relate to case outcome. Simmons and Freeman suggest, by implication, that psychiatric and other medical aspects are less important in determining case outcome than are the attitudes of relatives to whom the patient is returned.[1] Brown has found that the type of living arrangement to which patients were returned was the most significant factor in their success or failure.[2] Others have reasoned that the nature of hospital treatment procedures may be effective in keeping patients out of the hospital and functioning in the community. Related to these findings, although not precisely of the same nature, are the results obtained in incidence and prevalence studies such as those of Rennie and associates,[3] and Hollingshead and Redlich,[4] which emphasize socio-economic variables as determinative of who receives attention, the source of the treatment, the type of treatment, the duration of treatment, psychiatric diagnosis and eventually the re-entry into treatment.

This paper is wholly concerned with the extent to which psychiatric variables on the one hand and objective social attributes on the other are (a) predictive of success or failure in outcome, the latter defined as rehospitalization within six months after discharge, and (b) these same variables can foretell the level of patient functioning of those who remain in the community.

METHOD

The Columbus Psychiatric Institute and Hospital, an intensive therapy, short-term, heavily staffed institution discharged 376 female patients in the period December 1, 1958 through July 31, 1959. Of these released patients, 287 were studied intensively. Hospital and background data were also gathered for the remaining 89 cases who were excluded from the follow-up because they were either (a) returned to communities outside of the thirteen county area served by the hospital, or (b) transferred to another hospital within two weeks after initial hospital release.

The total failure rate for the entire population of 376 cases was 26 per cent including transfers to other hospitals; of the 287 study cases, 41 or 14 per cent were rehospitalized within six months after release.

In order to measure the level of patient functioning after discharge, trained and experienced psychiatric social workers conducted lengthy and structured interviews with the former patients and with a significant other, usually the husband, of each. The quality of posthospital patient performance was derived from responses to three scales in the interview schedules of the significant other. These scales consisted of (a) a 32 item index of psychological functioning taken in part from the Lorr Multidimensional Scale for Rating Psychiatric Patients, in part from a similar index utilized by Simmons and Freeman and in part from items developed by us, (b) a domestic functioning scale of nine items dealing with the patient's performance of routine duties customarily associated with the female role, and (c) a social participation index consisting of 11 items.[5]

Together these three indices comprised the total functioning of the patient in the community. On the basis of total scores on the combined index which ranged theoretically from 52 for the poorest possible functioner to 222 for the very best posthospital performer, patients were arbitrarily assigned to three functioning categories—low, medium and high.[6] Approximately one-third of the patients fell into each of these three classifications.

Independent evaluations, comparable to our psychological functioning index were also obtained. Two staff psychiatrists interviewed a total of 65 of the 287 patients. Their evaluations were found to be positively associated with those obtained from the significant others although the assessments of one psychiatrist were closer to those of the husbands than were the assessments of the second psychiatrist.[7]

In order to gather systematic information on the psychiatric and objective social attributes of the patients, a hospital record schedule form was developed which contained 88 different specific questions to be answered from the hospital records. When the records were incomplete on given items, patient charts and nursing and medical notes were consulted. Finally, when possible, comparable information was obtained in the interviews as another method of measuring reliability of patient and significant other responses and of confirming the hospital record information. Very little difference was found in contrasting the information contained in hospital records and in interview responses.

FINDINGS

Two general findings should be noted at the outset of this presentation. First, with only one exception, the various medical-psychiatric attributes of patients, including ward assignments, were less predictive of either rehospitalization or of posthospital level of functioning than were the social background attributes. Second, patients who were successful in remaining in the community but were classified as poor or low level functioners on the basis of their psychological and domestic performance and in their social participation were in some respects more similar to the rehospitalized patients than they were to the moderate or high level functioners. This would indicate that additional hospital returnees will probably be drawn from this category of patients.

MEDICAL-PSYCHIATRIC ATTRIBUTES AND CASE OUTCOME

Ward Assignment

Ward assignment ordinarily cannot be construed as a relevant psychiatric variable in case outcome. However, when patients are randomly assigned to three hospital wards on the basis of available bed space and are subjected to widely different ward treatment procedures, ward assignment becomes of necessity a meaningful medical factor in predicting outcome. Elsewhere we have tried to indicate that the three hospital wards housing female patients did in fact differ widely in their policies and practices with regard to patient care and treatment.[8] It was shown that these differences seemed to have little bearing on the overt behavior of the patients on the wards; indeed, that overt patient functioning did not differ from one ward to another. It is now possible to indicate that ward differences do not seem to be of much significance for outcome either. The data were analyzed in several ways. First, of all females released from the hospital, including transfers to other hospitals and out-of-area cases, the results indicate that the percentage of successful cases from each of the three wards was 74.2, 77.4 and 68.3 per cent respectively. Second, including only the interview cases, the comparable success percentages were 84.0, 83.0 and 88.6. In other words, once the transfers are excluded from consideration, the wards do not appreciably differ in their success and failure rates. Third, of the patients labelled as successful by dint of their ability to remain in the community at least six months, no differences, by ward, were found in their level of posthospital performance.

Admissions, Illness Duration, Length of Hospitalization

Rehospitalized patients could not be differentiated from successful patients nor successful cases from each other by functioning category in terms of their total number of previous admissions, illness duration preceding hospitalization or in their length of hospital stay. Two-thirds of all patients, regardless of outcome, had been first admissions. Illness duration prior to hospitalization varied from 5.4 years for the rehospitalized, 6.8 years for low functioners, 6.2 years for medium outcome cases and 5.6 years for high functioners. These differences were not statistically significant for any two of the groups or for all four groups considered simultaneously. Similarly, the length of hospitalization was greatest for the returnees (58.6 days on the average) and lowest for the low and moderate functioners (49 days). Nevertheless, even the most extreme differences in this respect were of no statistical consequence.

Diagnosis

There is little doubt that hospital diagnosis is of importance in predicting outcome. Both the returnees (19.5 per cent), and the low functioners (23.1 per cent) were clearly overrepresented among the patients diagnosed as indicating either acute or chronic brain syndromes. When the organic cases were eliminated from consideration, however, the percentages of psychotic and non-psychotic patients did not vary appreciably in the four outcome groups. Hence, a diagnosis of organic damage is an excellent predictor of poor outcome or rehospitalization. Unfortunately, other diagnoses fail to differentiate among outcome groups.

Addiction

As expected, favorable outcome seems to depend on the absence of addictions which are often related to mental disorder. There is, for example, a clear gradient among the outcome categories as regards alcohol and drug complicated cases. Of the returnees, 17.1 per cent had a history of alcoholism or drug addiction. The percentages for the low, medium and high functioners were 12.7, 12.3 and 3.9, respectively. In interviewing the significant others, it was found that a binge or chronic abuse of alcohol was not infrequently the major consideration of the significant other in returning the patient to this or another mental hospital.

Hospital Treatment

No significant differences, as already noted, were observed with regard to length of hospitalization and case outcome. Similarly, being subjected to electroconvulsive therapy did not seem to make any appreciable difference in outcome. In general, a smaller percentage of the poorer functioners and returnees received electro-shock treatment probably because of the greater frequency of organic cases among them, than of the moderate and high functioners. On the other hand, a greater percentage of returnees and low functioners (51 per cent) than of moderate and high functioners (34 per cent) were treated with drugs during the course of their hospitalization. The differences in drug treatment were statistically significant.

Release and Prognosis at Discharge

The type of discharge granted the patients in the four outcome categories did not vary significantly. The only observable discrepancy involved the greater proportion of trial visit discharges in the returnee group (26.8 per cent) as contrasted with the other three groups (14.6 per cent). Discharges contrary to medical advice (AMA) or without leave (AWOL) were lowest in the returnee and high functioning group (17.1 per cent) and highest for the moderate functioners (29.2 per cent).

The inability to accurately predict outcome is best demonstrated by the therapists' prognosis ratings of patients at discharge. Favorable prognoses were given 18.2 per cent of the returnees, 10.4 per cent of the low functioners, 24.6 per cent of the moderate functioners and 31.7 per cent of the high performers. On the other hand, the percentages of unimproved patients varied from 13.4 per cent for the low functioners to 7.9 per cent of the high functioners with only 9.1 per cent of the returnees being rated as unimproved.

Using therapists' ratings again, the four outcome groups were seen as being very similar in the extent of their impairment at admission and also at discharge. Whatever differences in these ratings did occur seemed to indicate the more severe impairment of the low performers. It is interesting to find that a third of all the patients were seen as being moderately or severely impaired at discharge and that the 43.7 per cent of the low functioners in this category was only very slightly above the entire group average in this respect.

Finally, data were also obtained on the posthospital treatment of the 287 patients. Approximately one-fifth of them in all outcome categories received no such posthospital services. Some 30 per cent either received additional outpatient care from our hospital or from private practitioners. Returnees most frequently availed themselves of this help (35.1 per cent) and low functioners did so in lesser numbers (17.9 per cent). On the other hand, three-fifths of the low functioners and two-fifths of the others received non-psychiatric medical attention after discharge.

OBJECTIVE SOCIAL ATTRIBUTES
AND CASE OUTCOME

Whereas the preceding section has indicated that the medical psychiatric variables, with the exception of diagnosis, are at best only very poor predictors of outcome, the results to follow indicate that a much stronger case can be made for the relation of objective social variables and outcome.

Age, Race, Religion and Rural-Urban Residence

Because of the relative homogeneity of the female patient population, minimal differences were found in age, race, religion or rural-urban residence of the patients. Patients in all four outcome groups were approximately 40 years of age, predominantly white (87 per cent), Protestant (81 per cent) and urban (83 per cent). On the other hand, marital status, family type, education and social class were related to case outcome.

Family Variables

Simmons and Freeman have previously shown that male ex-patients who are married are better functioners than patients in other marital categories.[9] They interpreted this to mean that wives are less tolerant of deviant behavior than are mothers, for example, and that they expect better performance from the former patients. The patient then is in a situation in which he either lives up to these expectations or is returned to the hospital. A second explanation, i.e., that the sicker patients generally fail to marry, has also been posited. Although these two explanations are not, by any means, incompatible, our data tend to support the former and refute the latter in this instance.

In order to test the thesis that married patients tend to be less ill at both admission and at discharge than are single or divorced and separated female patients, an analysis was made using (a) the therapists' ratings of patient psychiatric impairment at admission and at discharge and also their prognosis of outcome, and (b) four scales—the Schizo-phrenia, Depression, Psychiasthenia, and Hypochondriasis—of the MMPI, which is routinely administered at admission and discharge. A second analysis compared the MMPI results and the psychiatric impairment at admission and at discharge and prognosis of patients returning to one of eight types of living arrangement, e.g., conjugal, parental, sibling, child, non-kin, alone, etc.

The results of these analyses indicated that the degree of psychiatric disability at admission and at discharge as rated by the therapist as well as his prognosis of outcome was not at all related to the marital status of the patients or the type of household to which they were returned. The same held for the MMPI results.

Thus, marital status and living arrangements after dis-charge were not selective of differentially impaired patients. Yet these same variables were found to be very highly related to posthospital functioning. Married patients were found to be underrepresented among the low functioners and over-represented among the high performers. Parental families housed more of the low functioners and few of those rehos-pitalized. The specific details follow.

Less than half (46.8 per cent) of the low functioners, three-fifths of the moderate functioners and four-fifths of the high performers, were married. On the other hand, seven out of ten of the returnees also were married. Further, 43 per cent of the low, three-fifths of the moderate and three-fourths of the high performers were residing with their spouses as were 59 per cent of the returnees prior to rehos-pitalization. To make the same point another way, the returnees were very similar to the moderate and high func-tioners in being married and living with their spouses prior to rehospitalization.

Of the 24 patients who returned to their parents, few (8.3 per cent) were rehospitalized and a great many (41.7 per cent) were low performers. Of the 159 who were returned to their spouses more (14.5 per cent) were rehospitalized but far fewer (21.4 per cent) were poor performers. Of the 85 patients who lived in a non-parental, or non-conjugal house-hold or alone, a relatively high proportion (16.5 per cent) were rehospitalized and a high proportion (41.2 per cent) were performing poorly.

Not only will patients returned to a conjugal family perform better, but those returning to households with young children requiring care and attention and devoid of other adult females who can provide this care will do even better. Of the 182 patients who returned to a household in which there were no other adult females only 12.6 per cent were rehospitalized and an additional fourth were poor performers. On the other hand, significantly more of the patients returned to families having other adult females were both rehospitalized and functioned poorly. Again, Simmons and Freeman appear to be correct when they argue that patients do better when role replacements are unavailable.

Social Class Variables

The data indicate that class variables also seem to play a major role in outcome. Good posthospital performance appears to be related to relatively high educational attainment and socio-economic status. The fewest returnees came from ⁺he college educated group (9.4 per cent) and of those who had attended college, two-fifths proved to be high performers. The contrast between the college educated and those patients with only a grade school education was pronounced. Of the latter, 12.8 were rehospitalized, two-fifths functioned poorly and only one-fifth were among the high performers.

Finally, on the basis of a number of social class measures drawn from both the Warner Index of Status Characteristics and Hollingshead's Index of Social Position, low performers were observed to be drawn from the lower socio-economic segments of the hospital discharges, high performers from the highest socio-economic status segment, and returnees and moderate performers were representative of the middle hospital social status category.

DISCUSSION

The findings in this paper lend additional evidence to the proposition that the posthospital family milieu and the socio-economic status of the patient are fairly accurate predictors of case outcome. The hard psychiatric variables, on the other hand, seem to be relatively unimportant in assessing the recovery potential and posthospital performance of former mental patients.

The chief contribution of these data lies in their confirmation of hypotheses and conclusions previously suggested or reached by others. First, these results seem to substantiate the hypothesis that, when the degree of illness is controlled, familial variables seem to be extremely significant in determining case outcome. Married females are better posthospital performers than are single or divorced and separated women. Married women returned to a conjugal or nuclear family setting are superior functioners. The seemingly best posthospital functioners are married women, of relatively high socio-economic status residing in nuclear households, having relatively young children, and without other adult females to serve as role replacements. It is helpful, too, if they have been diagnosed as non-organic but it makes little difference whether they are classed as psychotic or non-psychotic.

The dynamics underlying the success of patients returned to this type of setting are suggested to be largely subjective (attitudinal) in nature. The significant others of patients in these households are likely to have high expectations for performance, the former patients themselves are also likely to expect more of themselves, their significant others are unlikely to be very tolerant of deviant behavior in the patient and greater external demands are likely to impinge upon them. These greater pressures for success and for a return to "normalcy" and to the fulfillment of the prerequisites of the female role are likely therefore to be translated into better posthospital performance.

One might even interpret these results to mean that the posthospital image by others of the patient as "sick" or not fully recovered or requiring special handling is self-defeating; that the redefinition of the patient as "well" and as one who should perform the routine female role(s) will result in superior functioning. The households containing the better functioners were, by their very nature, those in which the "sick" role could not be maintained.

If this interpretation, admittedly laced with a good deal of speculation but nonetheless consistent with previous findings is realistic, then certain practical consequences for patient care follow. Briefly, those would include minimizing the patients' "sick" role in the hospital by providing hospital tasks for patients to perform consistent with the extent of their disability, broadening of these responsibilities prior to release, and pre-release and posthospital counseling of family members as to the ability of the patient to assume certain obligations and responsibilities. It may even be that patients should be discouraged from returning to parental situations or to those in which role replacements are available. Before recommending these measures, however, a great deal of further inquiry into these matters is mandatory inasmuch as our data are as yet far too limited in scope and range for any but purely hypothetical suggestions to emerge.

The Abbotts

R. D. LAING AND A. ESTERSON

Maya is a tall, dark, attractive woman of twenty-eight. She is an only child. Until she was eight she lived with her mother and father, the manager of a general store. From then until fourteen she was an evacuee with an elderly childless couple and from fourteen to eighteen when she was first admitted to hospital, she was once again with her parents.

She has spent nine of her last ten years in West Hospital.

FROM *Sanity, Madness, and the Family*, Tavistock Publications, London, 1964, pp. 15–34. Reprinted by permission of the authors and the publisher.

CLINICAL PERSPECTIVE

Maya's 'illness' was diagnosed as paranoid schizophrenia. It appeared to come out of the blue. A report by a psychiatric social worker based on interviews with her mother and father described the onset in the following way:

Patient did not seem to be anything other than normal in her behaviour until about a month before her admission to hospital. She had of course been worrying about her school work, but the parents were used to this, and from past experience regarded her fears as quite groundless. One afternoon she came home from school and told her parents that the headmistress wished her to leave the school. Parents were immediately worried as they knew this was not right. Further, the patient reiterated this on other occasions. She then said that she could not sleep, and shortly afterwards became convinced that burglars were breaking into the house. A sedative was prescribed but the patient at first refused to take this. One night when she did so, she sat bolt upright in bed, and managed to stay awake in spite of the drug. She then decided her father was poisoning her, and one day ran out of the house and told a neighbour that her father was trying to poison her. Parents eventually found her and brought her home. She did not seem frightened of her father and discussed the matter quite calmly with him, but refused to be convinced that he was not trying to get rid of her. A doctor was called and advised that she have treatment immediately. Patient was more than willing to have treatment, and entered hospital as a voluntary patient.

Ten years later her parents gave us the same report.

In the past ten years her behaviour has given rise to clinical attributions that she had auditory hallucinations and was depersonalized; showed signs of catatonia; exhibited affective impoverishment and autistic withdrawal. Occasionally she was held to be 'impulsive'.

Expressed more phenomenologically, she experienced herself as a machine, rather than as a person: she lacked a sense of her motives, agency and intentions belonging together: she was very confused about her autonomous identity. She felt it necessary to move and speak with studious and scrupulous correctness. She sometimes felt that her thoughts were controlled by others, and she said that not she but her 'voices' often did her thinking.

In our account, as we are not approaching our study from

a clinical but from a social phenomenological perspective, we shall not be able to compartmentalize our inquiry in terms of clinical categories. Clinical signs and symptoms will become dissolved in the social intelligibility of the account that follows.

What we are setting out to do is to show that Maya's experiences and actions, especially those deemed most schizophrenic, become intelligible as they are seen in the light of her family situation. This 'situation' is not only the family seen by us from without, but the 'family' as experienced by each of its members from inside.

Our fundamental question is: to what extent is Maya's schizophrenic experience and behaviour intelligible in the light of the praxis and process of her family?

STRUCTURE OF INVESTIGATION

Our picture of this family is based on the following interviews.

Interviews	Occasions
Mother	1
Father	1
Daughter	2
Daughter and mother	29
Daughter and father	2
Mother and father	2
Mother, father, and daughter	8
	45

This represents fifty hours' interviewing, of which forty were tape-recorded.

THE FAMILY SITUATION

Mr. and Mrs. Abbott appear quiet, ordinary people. When Maya was eighteen Mrs. Abbott was described by a psychiatric social worker as "a most agreeable woman, who appeared to be friendly and easy to live with." Mr. Abbott had "a quiet manner but a kindly one." He seemed "a very sensible man, but less practical than his wife." There did not appear to be much that he would not do for his family. He had excellent health, and impressed the interviewer as "a very stable personality."

Maya was born when her mother was twenty and her father thirty.

When his daughter was born, Mr. Abbott had been reading of an excavation of a Mayan tomb. "Just the name for my little girl," he thought.

Mother and father agreed that until sent away from home at eight Maya had been her daddy's girl. She would wake him early in the morning and they would go swimming. She was always hand-in-hand with him. They sat close together at table, and he was the one to say prayers with her last thing at night. They frequently went for long walks together.

Apart from brief visits home, Maya lived away from her parents from eight until the age of fourteen. When she came home then to live permanently with them, they complained she was changed. She was no longer their little girl. She wanted to study. She did not want to go swimming, or to go for long walks with her father any more. She no longer wanted to pray with him. She wanted to read the Bible herself, by herself. She objected to her father expressing his affection for her by sitting close to her at meals. She wanted to sit further away from him. Nor did she want to go to the cinema with her mother. In the house, she wanted to handle things and to do things for herself, such as (mother's example) washing a mirror without first telling her mother.

These changes in Maya, mentioned by her parents retrospectively as the first signs of illness, seem to us to be ordinary expressions of growing up. What is of interest is the discrepancy between her parents' judgment of these developments and ours.

Maya conceived as her main difficulty, indeed her main task in life, the achievement of autonomy.

You should be able to think for yourself, work things out for yourself. I can't. People can take things in but I can't. I forget half the time. Even what I remember isn't true memory. You should be able to work things out for yourself.

Her parents appear to have consistently regarded with alarm all expressions of developing autonomy on Maya's part, involving necessarily efforts to separate herself from them and to do things on her own initiative. Her parents' alarm remains unabated in the present. For example, her mother objected to her ironing without supervision, although for the past year she had been working in a laundry without mishap. Mr. and Mrs. Abbott regarded their daughter's use of her own "mind," independently of them, as synonymous with "illness," and as a rejection of them. Her mother said:

I think I'm so absolutely centred on the one thing—it's well, to get her well—I mean as a child, and as a—teenager I could always sort out whatever was wrong or—do something about it, but it—but this illness has been so completely em—our relations have been different—you see Maya is er—instead of accepting everything—as if I said to her, er, "Black is black," she would have probably believed it, but since she's ill, she's never accepted anything any more. She's had to reason it out for herself, and if she couldn't reason it out herself, then she didn't seem to take *my* word for it—which of course is quite different to me.

"Since her illness," as they put it, she had become more "difficult." She did not "fit in" as she had done. The hospital had made her worse in this respect, although Maya felt that it had helped her to "use her own mind" more than before. Using one's own mind entails, of course, experiencing for oneself generally. What to Maya was "using my own mind," and "wanting to do things for myself," was to her parents "forwardness" and "brightness."

Until eighteen Maya studied hard, and passed all her exams. She took refuge, as she said, in her books, from what she called her parents' intrusions. Her parents' attitudes became highly equivocal, at one and the same time proud and patronizing, hurt in themselves and anxiously concerned for her. They said she was very clever, even "too clever perhaps." They thought she worked too hard. She was getting no enjoyment reading all the time, so she had to be dragged away from her reading. Her mother said:

We used to go to the pictures in those days and I used to say eh—and sometimes she'd say, "I don't think I should go to the pictures tonight, Mum, I think I should do some homework." And then I'd say to her, "Oh well, I'm disappointed," or that I'd made up my mind to go or something like that, or, "Well, I'll go on my own," and then she'd say, "All right, I will come." She really had to be forced to go out, most of the time.

When Maya said that her parents put difficulties in the way of her reading, they amusedly denied this. She insisted that she had wanted to read the Bible; they both laughed at the idea that they made this difficult for her, and her father, still laughing, said, "What do you want to read the Bible for anyway? You can find that sort of information much better in other books."

We shall now consider more closely certain recurring attributions made about Maya both by her parents and by psychiatrists.

For ten years she was described uniformly in psychiatric report after report as apathetic, withdrawn, lacking in affect, isolated, hostile, emotionally impoverished. Her parents also saw her in this way. She had been told by them so frequently since she was fourteen that she had no feelings, that one would have thought she would have been fairly inured to this attribution, yet she could still get flushed and angry when she was "accused" of it. For her part, she felt that she had never been given affection, nor allowed to show affection spontaneously, and that it was exasperation or frustration on this score that was the reason for much of what was called her impulsiveness—for instance, the incident that had occasioned her readmission to hospital eight years earlier, when she was said to have attacked her mother with a knife.

MAYA: Well why did I attack you? Perhaps I was looking for something, something I lacked—affection, maybe it was greed for affection.
MOTHER: You wouldn't have any of that. You always think that's soppy.
MAYA: Well, when did you offer it to me?
MOTHER: Well, for instance if I was to want to kiss you you'd say, "Don't be soppy."
MAYA: *But I've never known you let me kiss you.*

Maya made the point that her parents did not think of her, or "see" her as "a person," "as the person that I am." She felt frightened by this lack of recognition, and hit back at them as a means of self-defence. But this, of course, was quite bewildering to her parents, who could not grasp at any time any sense in this accusation. Maya insisted that her parents had no genuine affection for her because they did not know, and did not want to know, what she felt, and also that *she* was not allowed to express any spontaneous affection for *them*, because this was not part of "fitting in."

When Maya said that she had brightened up after having lost her feelings, her mother retorted, "Well, you were too bright already." This did not refer to any hypomanic quality about the girl, as there was none.

Another feature of her lack of feeling is illuminated by the issue of being taken seriously or not. As Maya said, her father

... often laughed off things that I told him and I couldn't see what he was laughing at. I thought it was very serious. Even when I was five, when I could understand, I couldn't see what he was laughing at. Both Father and Mother took sides against me.

I told Father about school and he used to laugh it off. If I told him about my dreams he used to laugh it off and tell me to take no notice. They were important to me at the time—I often got nightmares. He used to laugh them off. He played a lot with me as a child, but that's not the same.

Her mother complained to us that Maya did not want to understand her: her father felt the same way, and both were hurt that she would not tell them anything about herself.

Their response to this blow was interesting. They came to feel that Maya had exceptional mental powers, so much so that they convinced themselves *that she could read their thoughts*. For instance,

FATHER: If I was downstairs and somebody came in and asked how Maya was, if I immediately went upstairs, Maya would say to me, "What have you been saying about me?" I said, "Nothing." She said, "Oh yes you have, I heard you." Now it was so extraordinary that unknown to Maya I experimented myself with her, you see, and then when I'd proved it I thought, "Well I'll take Mrs. Abbott into my confidence," so I told her, and she said, "Oh don't be silly, it's impossible." I said, "All right, now when we take Maya in the car tonight I'll sit beside her and I'll concentrate on her. I'll say something, and you watch what happens." When I was sitting down she said, "Would you mind sitting on the other side of the car, I can't fathom Dad's thoughts." And that was true. Well, following that, one Sunday I said—it was winter—I said, "Now Maya will sit in the usual chair, and she'll be reading a book. Now you pick up a paper and I'll pick up a paper, and I'll give you the word and er . . . "—Maya was busy reading the paper, and er—I nodded to my wife, then I concentrated on Maya behind the paper. She picked up the paper—her em—magazine or whatever it was and went to the front room. And her mother said, "Maya where are you going? I haven't put the fire on." Maya said, "I can't understand—" no—"I can't get to the depth of Dad's brain. Can't get to the depth of Dad's mind."

Such experimentation has continued from before her first "illness" to the present, and came to light only after this investigation had been under way for over a year. In this light, it is only with the greatest difficulty that Maya's ideas of influence can continue to be seen as the effulgence of an individual pathological process, whether conceived as organic or psychic or both.

Clinically, she "suffered" from "ideas of influence." She recurred repeatedly to her feeling that despite herself she influenced others in untoward ways, and that others could and did influence her unduly, again despite her own struggles to counter this.

Now, in general, the nature of the reciprocal influences that persons do and can exert on one another is rather obscure. This is a realm where phantasy tends to generate fact. Certainly it would be easier to discuss Maya's preoccupation with this issue if clearer ideas existed among the sane population on what does and can happen in this respect.

Specifically, it will be very relevant to us to know answers to the following questions.

What influence did her mother and father feel that Maya actually had on them?

What influence did they feel they could or did have, or ought to have had, on her?

What influence did they try to have on her?

What influence did they assume that one person could have on another, especially by action from a distance, and particularly by prayer, telepathy, or thought-control—the media that worried Maya most?

Without answers to such questions, no one could start to evaluate and elucidate Maya's 'delusions' of reciprocal influence. This principle necessarily holds, it seems to us, for every instance of such delusions.

In this case ideas of influence become socially intelligible when we remember that her parents *were* actively trying to influence her, that they believed that she could tell their thoughts, and that they experimented with her and denied to her that they did so. Further, while ascribing these remarkable powers to Maya, they believed, without any sense of contradiction, that she did not even know what she thought or did herself.

Maya's accusations that her mother and father were "influencing" her in some way were "laughed off" by them, and it is not surprising, therefore, that at home especially she was irritable, jumpy, and confused. It was only in the course of our investigation, as we have said, that they admitted to her what they had been doing.

MAYA: Well I mean you shouldn't do it—it's not natural.

FATHER: I don't do it—I didn't do it—I thought, "Well I'm doing the wrong thing, I won't do it."

MAYA: I mean the way I react would show it's wrong.

FATHER: And there was a case in point a few weeks back—she fancied one of her mother's skirts.

MAYA: I didn't—I tried it on and it fitted.

FATHER: Well they had to go to a dressmaker—the dressmaker was recommended by someone. Mrs. Abbott went for it, and she said, "How much is that?" The woman said, "Four shillings"—Mrs. Abbott said, "Oh no, it must have cost you more than that." So she said, "Oh well, your husband did me a good turn a few years back and I've never repaid him." I don't know what it was. Mrs. Abbott gave more of course. So when Maya came home she said, "Have you got the skirt, Mum?" She said, "Yes, and it cost a lot of money too, Maya"—Maya said, "Oh you can't kid me—they tell me it was four shillings."

MAYA: No, seven I thought it was.

FATHER: No, it was four you said—exactly—and my wife looked at me and I looked at her—So if you can account for that—I can't.

An idea of reference that she had was that something she could not fathom was going on between her parents, seemingly about her.

Indeed there was. When they were all interviewed together, her mother and father kept exchanging with each other a constant series of nods, winks, gestures, knowing smiles, so obvious to the observer, that he commented on them after twenty minutes of the first such interview. They continued, however, unabated and denied.

The consequence, so it seems to us, of this failure by her parents to acknowledge the validity of similar comments by Maya, was that Maya could not know when she was perceiving or when she was imagining things to be going on between her parents. These open yet unavowed non-verbal exchanges between father and mother were in fact quite public and perfectly obvious. Much of what could be taken to be paranoid about Maya arose because she mistrusted her own mistrust. She could not really believe that what she thought she saw going on was going on. Another consequence was that she could not easily discriminate between actions not usually intended or regarded as communications, e.g. taking off spectacles, blinking, rubbing nose, frowning, and so on, and those that are—another aspect of her paranoia. It was just those actions, however, that were used as signals between her parents, as "tests" to see if Maya would pick them up, but an essential part of this game the parents played was that, if commented on, the rejoinder would be an amused, "What do you mean?," "What wink?," and so on.

In addition to attributing to her various wonderful powers, her parents added further to her mystification by telling her she could not, or did not, think, remember, or do what she did think, remember, and do.

It is illuminating to compare in some detail what she and her mother had to say about the supposed attack on her mother that had precipitated her readmission to hospital (see p. 135 above).

According to her mother, Maya attacked her for no reason. It was the result of her illness coming on again. Maya said she could not remember anything about it. Her mother continually prompted Maya to try to remember.

Maya once said, however, that she could remember the occasion quite clearly. She was dicing some meat. Her mother was standing behind her, telling her how to do things right, and that she was doing things wrong as usual. She felt something was going to snap inside unless she acted. She turned round and brandished the knife at her mother, and then threw it on the floor. She did not know why she felt like that. She was not sorry for what had happened, but she wanted to understand it. She said she had felt quite well at the time: she did not feel that it had to do with her "illness." She was responsible for it. She had not been told to act like that by her "voices." The voices, she said, were her own thoughts, anyway.

Our construction is that the whole episode might have passed unnoticed in many households as an expression of ordinary exasperation between daughter and mother.

We were not able to find one area of Maya's personality that was not subject to negations of different kinds.

For instance, she thinks she started to imagine "sexual things" when she came home at the age of fourteen. She would lie in bed wondering whether her parents had sexual intercourse. She began to get sexually excited, and to masturbate. She was very shy, however, and kept away from boys. She felt increasingly irritated at the physical presence of her father. She objected to his shaving in the same room while she had breakfast. She was frightened that her parents knew that she had sexual thoughts about them. She tried to tell them about this, but they told her *she did not have any thoughts of that kind*. She told them she masturbated *and they told her that she did not*. What happened then is of course inferred, but *when she told her parents in the presence of the interviewer that she still masturbated, her parents simply told her that she did not!*

As she recalls, when she was fifteen she began to feel that her father was causing these sexual thoughts, and that both parents were trying to influence her in some queer way. She intensified her studies, burying herself in her books, but she began to hear what she was reading in her head, and she began to hear her own thoughts. She was now struggling hard to think clearly any thoughts of her own. Her thoughts thought themselves audibly in her head: her vocal cords spoke her voice, her mind had a front and a back part. Her movements came from the front part of her mind. They just happened. She was losing any sense of being the agent of her own thoughts and words.

Not only did both her parents contradict Maya's memory, feelings, perceptions, motives, intentions, but they made attributions that were themselves curiously self-contradictory, and, while they spoke and acted as though they knew better than Maya what she remembered, what she did, what she imagined, what she wanted, what she felt, whether she was enjoying herself or whether she was tired, this control was often maintained in a way which was further mystifying.

For instance, on one occasion Maya said that she wanted to leave hospital, and that she thought her mother was trying to keep her in hospital, even though there was no need for her to be an in-patient any more. Her mother replied:

I think Maya is—I think Maya recognizes that—er—whatever she wanted really for her good, I'd do—wouldn't I—Hmm? (no answer)—No reservations in any way—I mean if there are any changes to be made I'd gladly make them—unless it was absolutely impossible.

Nothing could have been further from what Maya recognized at that moment. But one notes the many mystifying qualifications in the statement. Whatever Maya wanted is qualified most decisively by "really" and "for her own good." Mrs. Abbott, of course, was arbiter (i) of what Maya recognized, (ii) of what Maya "really" wanted, in contrast to what *she* might *think* she wanted, (iii) of what was for her own good, (iv) of what was a reservation or a change, (v) of what was possible.

Maya sometimes commented fairly lucidly on these mystifications. But this was much more difficult for her to do than for us. Her difficulty was that she could not know when to trust or mistrust her own perceptions and memory or her mother and father.

The close investigation of this family reveals that her parents' statements to her about her, about themselves, about what they felt she felt they felt, and even about what could directly be seen and heard, could not be trusted.

Maya *suspected* this, but her parents regarded just such suspicions as her illness, and they told her so. She often therefore doubted the validity of her own suspicions: sometimes she denied delusionally what they said, sometimes she invented a story to cling to, for instance, that she had been in hospital when she was eight—the occasion of her first separation from them.

It is not so surprising that Maya tried to withdraw into her own world, although feeling at the same time most painfully that she was not an autonomous person. However, she felt that in order to win some measure of separateness from her parents, she required to cultivate what she called "self-possession." This had various ramifications.

> If I weren't self-possessed I'd be nowhere, because I'd be mixed up in a medley of other things.

As we have seen, however, it was just this attempt at autonomy that her parents saw as her "illness," since it entailed that she did not "fit in" with them, and was "difficult," "forward," "too bright," "too proud," and found fault with them.

Maya tried to explain herself in these terms:

> I emphasize people's faults to regain my self-possession.
> I can't fit in properly with people: it's not pride.
> Mother is always picking on me. She's always getting at me. She's always trying to teach me how to use my mind. You can't tell a person how to use their mind against their will. It has always been like that with Mother. I resent it.

But at other times she doubted the validity of this impression. She said:

> She doesn't pick on me, but that's how I look at it. That's how I react to it. I've got to calm myself. I always feel I've got to pick back at her— to stand up and get my own back—get back my self-possession.

She would feel that her mother and father were forcing their opinions on her, that they were trying to "obliterate" her mind. But she had been taught to suppose that this was a mad thing to think, that this was what her "illness" was.

So, she sought temporary refuge in her own world, her private world, her shell. To do this, however, was to be "negative," in her parents' jargon: "withdrawn," in psychiatric parlance.

When she was not putting up as belligerent a self-defensive

front as she could muster, Maya would admit that she was very unsure of her own faculties. Things were not always real.

I was never allowed to do anything for myself so I never learned to do things. The world doesn't seem quite real. If you don't do things then things are never quite real.

Change disturbed her precarious sense of identity.

I don't know how to deal with the unexpected. That's why I like things neat and tidy. Nothing unexpected can happen then.

But this neatness and tidiness had to come from herself, not be imposed by her parents' "correctness" or "precision."

I used to think it a threat when I was younger, when I didn't have the freedom to act otherwise, but I can act otherwise now: but their correctness makes me want to understand why they are so correct, why they do things as they do, and why I am like I am.

She repeatedly disclaimed any feelings of her own, and any interest in other people's feelings.

Mother is a person that I lived with. I don't feel any more strongly than that. If something happened to her I should miss her and I should keep on thinking about her, but it wouldn't make any difference to the way I go on. I haven't any deep feelings. I'm just not made that way.

But she certainly knew what fear was. For instance, when an aunt shouted at her recently.

I felt just—I've often seen the cat shrink and it felt like that inside me.

She herself disclaimed being the agent of her own thoughts, largely, it seems, to evade criticism and invalidation.

I don't think, the voices think.

They echoed her reading or they made "criticisms" of people she was terrified to make in her own person.

Just as not she but the voices thought, so not she but her body acted.

The whole lot is out of my control.

She had given up trying to "make out" what her parents or anyone else was up to.

> I can only see one side of the question—the world through my eyes and I can't see it through anyone else's eyes, like I used to.

This repudiation of any desire to "put herself into" others was partly a defensive tactic, but it was also an expression of the fact that she was genuinely at a loss.

> I find it hard to hold down a job because I don't know what is going on in other people's minds, and they seem to know what I'm thinking about.
> I don't like being questioned on anything because I don't always know what other people are thinking.
> I can't make out your kind of life. I don't live in your world. I don't know what you think or what you're after, and I don't want to (addressing her mother).

Her parents could see Maya's attempts at "self-possession" only as due to "a selfish nature," "greed," "illness," or "lack of feeling."

Thus when Maya tried to get into her own shell, to live in her own world, to bury herself in her books (to use her expressions), her mother and father felt this, as we have seen, as a terrible blow. The only time in our interviews when Mrs. Abbott began to cry was when, having spoken of her own mother's death, she said that Maya did not want to understand her, because she was only interested in her own problems.

Mrs. Abbott persistently reiterated how much she hoped and prayed that Maya would remember anything if it would help the doctors to get to the bottom of her illness. But she felt she had to tell Maya repeatedly that she (Maya) could not "really" remember anything, because (as she explained to us) Maya was always ready to pretend that she was not really ill.

She frequently questioned Maya about her memory in general, in order (from her point of view) to help her to realize that she was ill, by showing her at different times either that she was amnesic, or that she had got her facts wrong, or that she only imagined she remembered what she thought she remembered because she had heard about it from her mother or father at a later date.

This "false" but "imaginary" memory was regarded by Mrs. Abbott with great concern. It also worried and confused Maya.

Mrs. Abbott finally told us (not in Maya's presence) that she prayed that Maya would never remember her "illness" because she (Mother) thought it would upset her (the daughter) to do so. Indeed, she felt this so strongly, that it would be "kindest" if Maya never remembered her "illness," even if it meant she had to remain in hospital!

A curious and revealing moment occurred when she was speaking of how much it meant to her that Maya should get well. Mrs. Abbott had said that for Maya to get "well" would mean that she would once more be "one with her." She usually spoke of her devotion to Maya as laying claim to gratitude from her, but now she spoke differently. She had been saying that maybe Maya was frightened to "get all right." She recalled a "home truth" a friend had given her recently about her relation to Maya.

She said to me, you know, "Well, you can't live anyone's life for them—you could even be punished for doing it"—And I remember thinking, "What a dreadful thing to think," but afterwards I thought she might be right. It struck me very forcibly. She said to me, "You get your life to live, and that's *your* life—you can't and you mustn't live anybody's life for them." And I thought at the time, "Well what a dreadful thing to think." And then afterwards I thought, "Well, it's probably quite right."

This insight, however, was fleeting.

In the foregoing we have examined various "signs" and "symptoms" that are almost universally regarded in the psychiatric world as "caused" by a disease, i.e., an organic pathological process, probably largely determined by genetic-constitutional factors, which destroys or impairs the organism's capacity to experience and to act in various ways.

In respect of depersonalization, catatonic and paranoid symptoms, impoverishment of affect, autistic withdrawal and auditory hallucinations, confusion of "ego boundaries," it seems to us, in this case, more likely that they are the outcome of her interexperience and interaction with her parents. They seem to be quite in keeping with the social reality in which she lived.

It might be argued as regards our historical reconstructions that her parents might have been reacting in an abnormal way to the presence of an abnormal child. The data hardly support this thesis. Her mother and father reveal plainly, *in the present*, that what they regard most as symptoms of illness are what we regard as developing personalization, realization, autonomy, spontaneity, etc. On their own testimony, everything points to this being the case in the past as well. Her parents felt as stress not so much the loss but the development of her self.

APPENDIX

List of some of the disjunctive attributions and perspectives of mother, father, and daughter, most but not all of which have been discussed above. (Condensed from tape-recordings.)

Daughter's View	*View of Mother and Father*
She said that:	Parents said that:
Blackness came over her when she was eight.	It did not. Her memory is at fault. She was imagining this. This showed a "mental lapse."
She was emotionally disturbed in the years eight to fourteen.	She was not.
She started to masturbate when she was fifteen.	She did not.
She masturbates now.	She does not.
She had sexual thoughts about her mother and father.	She did not.
She was worried over her examinations.	She never worried over examinations because she always passed them, and so

Daughter's View	*View of Mother and Father*
	she had no need to worry. She was too clever and worked too hard. Besides, she could not have worried because they would have known.
Her mother and father tried to stop her reading.	Nonsense: *and* She had to be torn away from her books. She was reading too much.
Her mother and father were trying to influence her in some ways.	Nonsense: *and* Attempts to influence her through prayer, telepathy, thought-control.
She was not sure whether they could read her mind.	They thought they knew her thoughts better than she did.
She was not sure whether she could read their minds.	They felt she had telepathic powers, etc.
She could remember the "attack" on her mother quite clearly but could not explain it.	She could not remember it.
She was responsible for it.	She was not responsible for it. She was ill. It was part of her illness that she said she could remember this, and that she said she was responsible for it.
Her mother was responsible for her being sent away as a result of this episode.	This was not so. She (mother) did not even know she was going to hospital when the doctor drove them both away in his car.
Her parents said they wanted her to get well, but they did not want her to get well.	It was her illness that made her say things like that.
Getting well was equivalent	There is nothing for her to

Daughter's View	*View of Mother and Father*
to: understanding why she attacked her mother; being able to use her own mind with self-confidence.	understand. Her illness made her do it.
	Since she has been ill Maya has been much more difficult—i.e.:
If you are not allowed to do things yourself things become unreal.	(i) she wanted to do things herself without first asking or telling them.
	(ii) she did not take their word for anything. She tried to make up her own mind about everything.
She could not always be sure whether she imagined feelings, or whether she really did have them.	(iii) she tried to remember things even in her childhood. And if she could not remember, she tried to imagine what happened.
	She should forget them.
She did not know why she had nightmares.	"I don't think dreams are any part of me. They are just things that happen to me."
	(Mother)

A Review of *Sanity, Madness, and the Family*

JOHN K. WING

Dr. Laing and Dr. Esterton have written one of those useful books which force the open minded reader to reconsider his preconceptions and discover his prejudices. It is refreshing to see the old problems of schizophrenia being examined in a new context, and stimulating to undertake the intellectual exercises involved in continuing the author's argument to its logical conclusion. But this is also a disappointing book because one has the feeling throughout that good material is being wasted. Dr. Laing summarized his data and presented his views in NEW SOCIETY of 16 April and I will confine myself, therefore, to a discussion of the issues which the book raises for me, a research worker in the same field.

Very briefly, the theory assumes that schizophrenia is not an illness in the classical medical sense but a mode of living, comprehensible as the only possible method of coping with a family situation which would otherwise be intolerable. The authors do not seriously consider the strong case that can be made for the conventional viewpoint and they do not set out the essential particulars which, for them, differentiate an "illness" from a "mode of living." This is reserved for a later volume, and the present work is presented mainly as an exercise in method.

The material published so far consists of a series of ex-

FROM *New Society* 84 (May 7, 1964) 23–24. Reprinted by permission of the author and publisher.

tracts from interviews with various combinations of family members, summaries and descriptions of other parts of the interviews, and a linking commentary. The aim of the book is to enable the reader to share the authors' understanding of how the family relationships, seen as a whole, contain the schizophrenic patient as a necessary part. The interviews, most of which were recorded on tape, concerned eleven patients and totalled from 14 to 50 hours per family.

The study, therefore, falls into that large group of investigations of the family circumstances of schizophrenic patients, in which a great deal of material, collected from a few people, is used as the basis for a very complicated theoretical formulation. The claim made by the authors is not a modest one:

In this book, we believe that we show that the experience and behaviour of schizophrenics is much more socially intelligible than has come to be supposed by most psychiatrists. We have tried in each single instance to answer the question: to what extent is the experience and behaviour of that person, who has already begun a career as a diagnosed "schizophrenic" patient, intelligible in the light of the praxis and process of his or her family nexus? We believe that the shift of point of view that these descriptions both embody and demand has an historical significance no less radical than the shift from a demonological to a clinical viewpoint 300 years ago.

This belief cannot properly be examined until the second volume is available but it is legitimate, at this stage, to consider in some detail the methods used by the authors to collect, analyze and present their data, in order to discover whether they have taken every precaution possible to prevent their own preconceptions from biasing their results.

It is not only would-be scientists who have to show that they are concerned to discover the truth, rather than simply to expound their favourite theory whatever the circumstances. The instructions of the London Missionary Society to its field workers (who included Livingstone) contained the following injunction:

State freely your trials and difficulties, as well as your encouragements and success. . . . Maintain that sacred control over your imagination and feelings which, while it shall not allow you to withhold what is due to the Directors and the friends of the Society, shall preserve you from a mode of representation adapted to mislead, by producing an impression in any respect at variance with truth and fact. . . .

Karl Popper said that if scientific objectivity depended only on the impartiality of individual scientists, "we should have to say goodbye to it."

Fortunately, there are techniques through which bias can be reduced, even in the presentation of a complex study of family relationships. For example, a systematic summary of important data can be given. This the authors barely attempt. There is no standard social or personal history, even where some element in it is crucial to the argument, and the demographic data given are minimal. The clinical material is reminiscent of mental hospital case records of the scantiest kind. Thus the social situations discussed, and the clinical phenomena which are supposed to arise out of them, are highly selected, and the reader can only guess at what has been left out.

Another technique for reducing bias and for making the study repeatable is to lay down standards of interviewing. This again the authors do not do. They give no information about how they conducted their sessions with family members, though it is clear that they allowed themselves to ask leading questions. Presumably the interviews were guided mainly by the necessity for reaching an understanding of the symptoms. This process must necessarily have been a personal one. Even so, it would help if, instead of giving only illustrations which made their point, the authors sorted their material into categories, each representing some family mechanism which they thought important and could define, and then selected illustrations at random from these so that the reader could judge for himself the quality of the data, the appropriateness of the sorting and the relevance of the material to their argument. As it is, the reader has no check on what they are doing and must take it entirely on trust. This is a dangerous situation, as Popper pointed out.

The process of categorization is, of course, a crude form of measurement. The authors suggest that the parents are unduly rigid in applying discipline, in toilet training, in limiting their children's normal social or sexual activities and in restricting or preventing their ability to become individuals in their own right. All these factors are susceptible of some degree of definition and of quantification. The same is true of the process called by Dr. Laing "mystification." This consists in the parent saying one thing while doing another, and expecting the child to react to what is said rather than to what is done. This almost universal technique for dealing with difficult situations (or, more bluntly, for covering up dirty work) is said to be very characteristic of the relations between parents and children who later are diagnosed as schizophrenic. This is the point at which some control families would be very useful. In 14-50 hours of interviewing with members of average families it is scarcely conceivable that many "abnormalities" would not be discovered. How common are the interesting factors described by Dr. Laing and Dr. Esterson? There is no means of knowing without some quantification, however crude, and without such a comparison it is surely unreasonable of the authors to be so confident of their interpretations?

Let us suppose, however, that specific abnormalities *had* been shown to occur with unusual regularity in families where there is a schizophrenic member. The next step would be to determine whether the presence of the patient caused the abnormalities, or whether the abnormalities caused the patient's condition. The authors assume the latter but they do not really discuss the problem. To take an example—if a mongol child were born into a family whose relationships had been passed as satisfactory by Dr. Laing, would any of his specific factors subsequently appear, provoked by the abnormality in the child? The family relationships would certainly be irrevocably altered if the child stayed at home. If schizophrenia is an illness, or group of illnesses, the first manifestations of which begin some time during childhood, the characteristics of the interactions between family members many years later, when the condition had become florid and recognizable, might be explicable in these terms. Another way of gaining useful information would be to study the interactions between family members when one of the *parents* was schizophrenic or otherwise mentally abnormal.

If the specific features were present the children could be followed into adult life to see whether they themselves became schizophrenic.

Yet other control techniques are possible. One of the most obvious is to study the brothers and sisters of schizophrenics. As children they have been exposed to the same sorts of family relationships and many will have been caught up in the "mystification" process. Some of them will have found the situation intolerable and they should therefore presumably become schizophrenic themselves. We know, of course, that the prevalence of schizophrenia is higher among these siblings than in the general population, but it is still only about 14 per cent. The vast majority do not develop schizophrenia. Why not? Some utilize non-schizophrenic methods of escape from an impossible situation (leaving home, suicide, crime, drug addiction, alcoholism, neurosis). Why?

Clearly one cannot criticize Dr. Laing and Dr. Esterson for not having carried out this series of studies. However, it *is* possible to devise situations in which some of the authors' hypotheses could be tested, and which might well show them to be wrong. The more such tests were successfully passed, the stronger would be the authors' case. Meanwhile, one must be grateful for the ideas put forward in this book and for a bold challenge to orthodox doctrines. For these, at any rate, the book is worth reading, and is to be recommended.

PART III

Social-Psychological
Aspects of Psychiatric
Treatment

This section begins with an examination of the ambiguous meaning of the psychiatric symptom by the psychiatrist Jules Coleman. In the second article, another psychiatrist, Jerome Frank, describes the social-psychological dimensions of psychotherapy. Bursten and D'esopo delineate a particular portion of the social environment of illness, the expectations that some persons should remain in the "sick role." Wing's article finally demonstrates some of the effects of prolonged hospitalization on the patient's motivation and other attitudes. All of these articles suggest that in some of its aspects, psychiatric treatment is a purely social and psychological process.

Social Factors Influencing the Development and Containment of Psychiatric Symptoms

JULES V. COLEMAN

In considering how psychiatric symptoms are influenced by social factors, I shall take the symptom itself as a point of departure, and discuss how it is regarded and what is generally included in the category of psychiatric symptoms. I shall point out the variability of symptom manifestations in duration and intensity, and discuss the relation of symptoms to distress and illness. I shall consider the assimilation of the symptom to ego control, whereby it becomes itself an ego-syntonic aspect of personality function. Finally, I shall discuss the use of symptoms in the context of social experience, and the extent to which symptoms serve as indicators and expressions of social disorganization.

Psychiatric symptoms serve a variety of functions, among which are the following: (1) *Retrospective or historical*, in the sense that they express and record certain kinds of resolution of problems and conflicts experienced by the individual in his previous history; (2) *Adaptive*, in that they have a significant role in the person's relationship system; (3) *Assimilative*, in that they come to be represented in the character structure; (4) *Restitutive*, in that they serve a

AN unpublished paper given at the *First International Congress of Social Psychiatry*. Published by permission of the author.

bridging function in restoring lost accesses to the real world; and (5) *Communicative*, in that they convey information to others about certain facets of the person's self-feelings.

Retrospective or historical symptoms occur in the neuroses particularly, and represent compromises between regressive strivings and the demands of the environment. They are prominent in such conditions as the phobias, hysterias, and obsessional neuroses. If symptoms persist, they tend to be adapted to the requirements of everyday living. A phobic, for example, will go to considerable lengths to adapt his doings to his necessary avoidances, but once the pattern of avoidance is established, it becomes an end in itself and is not necessarily experienced as illness or even as inconvenience.

In symptomatic behavior one observes the clearest examples of symptom assimilation, in which neurotic character distortions impose their own imperatives on the person's relations with others, leading to "as if" assumptions in the areas of distorted relationship. The person acts "as if" others were criticizing him, or devaluating him, or depriving him of what is emotionally rightfully his, and so on, but also often assumes that this is the way it is, and there can be no other way. The restitutive function of symptoms is seen in psychotic reactions. Finally, the symptom is a form of communication to others, having as its special purpose to invite responses appropriate to the person's symptom pattern.

There are at least two prominent attitudes among psychiatrists toward psychiatric symptoms. They are regarded as evidence of disturbance or illness, undesirable by definition, and requiring treatment and eradication, if possible. At the same time, it is also recognized, mainly under the influence of psychoanalysis, that a symptom is a meaningful expression of underlying personal problems, and that treatment should be directed towards the understanding and relief of these problems. It is of interest that both views are generally maintained at the same time, i.e. that symptoms have no significance except in relation to the problems they reveal, and also that symptoms are undesirable in themselves.

We use the term "symptom" as it is generally used in psychiatry, to include all psychopathological manifestations, e.g., compromise formations as in hysteria, regressed behavior as in the infantilisms, inhibitions of a special and general nature, behavior based on projection and denial, and psychotic mental processes such as hallucinations and delusions. Symptoms show great variation in their duration, persistence and modifiability. Certain symptoms, like the phobias, have a strong tendency to persist in their original form, moving to the foreground or receding from view as circumstances change. Other manifestations, like the thought disorders and affect distortion in schizophrenia become so completely identified with personality functioning that we feel justified in referring to a "schizophrenic personality," by which we mean a person whose functional integrity is intact, but who reveals expressive peculiarities readily perceived by the trained observer. Likewise, we refer to "infantile," "hysterical" or "compulsive" personalities, again not suggesting thereby that the person is ill, but that he reveals character traits which apparently derive from the transformation of symptoms. Finally, there are persons who develop symptoms in periods of crisis, and these may come and go (anxiety attacks, depressions, psychosomatic symptoms like peptic ulcer or asthma), their duration and persistence depending on the individual and his crises. With all types of symptoms, persons may function well until they meet an untried, stressful situation, or until their accustomed situations undergo significant change in the degree of social support, when an "acute episode" begins to emerge. Stressful changes in life experience are closely related to symptom fluctuation and variability.

Transiency of symptoms has been particularly observed in relation to the periodic crises which appear in the course of childhood development. However, even among adults, the great tendency of symptoms to resolve spontaneously has been noted among patients applying for outpatient psychiatric treatment. It has been found that many who for one reason or another do not receive treatment report after a time that their symptoms have cleared spontaneously, so that they no longer feel any need for the care they had originally applied for.[1, 2]

Here one needs to assess the relation between reaching

out for help and the presence of symptoms. One might suggest that persons seek help not because they are disturbed by their symptoms but because they experience feelings of distress. The symptom then becomes a "ticket of admission" to a treatment facility. It is also likely that what undergoes spontaneous remission is the state of distress, the symptoms automatically receding to the background of awareness of the patient begins to feel better. The evidence for the persistence of at least certain kinds of symptoms among adults is, however, very strong. Studies of persons diagnosed as schizophrenic and phobic at our clinic over 20 years ago indicated that they still retained many of the symptoms which had first brought them to the clinic.[3, 4] A study by Ernst[5] on the prognosis of the neuroses likewise indicated a strong tendency for symptoms to persist, either in their original form or by transformation to other symptom manifestations. Anxiety states, obsessive-compulsive symptoms, hypochondriacal manifestations, and neurasthenic complaints all showed persistence over decades in patients who had originally been seen in a psychiatric outpatient clinic.

There is, of course, no way to evaluate the significance of symptom formation and its relation to distress states in persons who do not apply for psychiatric care. The fact of the matter is that our entire scheme of classification of psychiatric symptoms is medical in tradition and practice. Whenever we examine behavioral deviance under other than medical auspices, we still tend to reduce it to symptom categories. A recent population study by Srole[6] and his associates found that only 18 percent of the persons studied were free of symptoms, by their own reports. In this study, it was found that 23.4 percent of the sample population were considered to be suffering from psychiatric disability. Because studies of this kind include a large number of persons in their sample, their results are difficult to evaluate since the investigation in depth of each individual is not possible. Furthermore, there are in any case no very reliable criteria for evaluating either good health or psychiatric disability in any systematic way.

In any event, there are ample indications that psychiatric symptoms are widespread in the population, perhaps even ubiquitous, and that few escape them. If symptoms are so common, they may well serve a function in the social adaptation of the individual. One might think of a symptom as a specialized form of adaptation, serving the purpose of reducing tension by effecting tolerable compromises among competing inner drives, and between drives and external stresses. The symptom is also the specific expression of distress appropriate to a particular person. Although many symptoms have a tendency to persist, they maintain fluctuating levels of intensity. Periods or episodes in which symptoms come into heightened awareness follow a curve of great irregularity; they are dependent upon the vicissitudes of circumstance and on the stresses to which the person is particularly vulnerable.

The symptom not only represents a means of dealing with unresolved intrapsychic tensions or conflicts, it is also a mode of communication. It imparts to others information about the person's view of his limitations, handicaps, or burdens, and the social restrictions associated with them. In other words, symptoms not only express a system of adaptive limitation, but also convey to others how the adaptive capacity is impaired, as well as its justification. In all of this, the symptom is not generally presented by the subject as an expression of illness, although it may be, but as an adaptive limitation or a personal handicap, usually transient or idiosyncratic in nature. This differs from the medical view of illness in which there is emphasis on onset and progression. Even in psychiatry, mental illness is often regarded as a predetermined "unfolding" process, often in the direction of progressive deterioration.

Aside from the presence of symptoms, the sense of being psychiatrically ill appears to be a highly complicated process related to social sanction, situational stresses, and social cohesion, as well as to individual vulnerability, and issues of personal values and identity. Deviance in behavior and thought occurs universally in all contexts of human experience. In day by day living, people are accustomed to correct for deviances they perceive in others, if the behavior is consensually average (i.e. if it is roughly consistent with social expectations). On the other hand, when we look at behavior in a psychiatric setting, i.e. when we are studying others as patients, we tend to give undue prominence to deviances which may not have the connotation of illness when seen in the perspective of the individual's current life pattern, or when weighed in the balance of his integrative ego function. Whether a person is psychiatrically ill, moreover, depends to some extent, although of course not entirely, on whether he thinks that he is; it is certainly a prerequisite in motivating application for psychiatric assistance.

A major source of difficulty in psychiatric diagnosis and evaluation is that symptoms are considered to be pathological manifestations regardless of the context in which they appear. In themselves, however, symptoms are neither normal nor abnormal; they derive significance only in relation to the individual's ecological system. Symptoms may serve a useful function in maintaining an individual's ecological balance. It is only when this balance is disturbed that the person reaches out for help, but psychiatric treatment is only one relatively minor resource among many which are socially available in restoring ecological balance. For this reason, the so-called "acute episode" is undoubtedly of much greater occurrence than would be gathered from an examination of the statistics of psychiatric facilities. Moreover, since many persons seek psychiatric help for reasons which are not necessarily associated with a sense of being ill, or with an acute episode, but for other reasons, such as refuge, retreat, loneliness, unhappiness, distress and despair, it is likely that cases in treatment are not always justifiably classified as psychiatric problems.

By and large, it seems reasonable to assume that social forces and group influences are inherently supportive and stabilizing of human behavior, and that primary stabilizing influences are inherent in the way society is organized. It may also be assumed that each society provides institutions which pattern emotional and personal expressions, as well as behavior in general, and that societies have their own structured ways of providing learning experiences during the developmental period, which indoctrinate social responses of supportive value to the individual.

The developmental process in childhood provides a means

not only of integrating growth gains but also of coping with characteristic disturbances of equilibrium. These are learning experiences. The ego finds solutions to these recurring disturbances in a way which takes into account the social situation as well as the emerging personality and its coping capacities. A basic principle of ego functioning is that equilibrium must be restored at whatever level is feasible, i.e. an effort at stabilization must be made even if it means that the individual has to live with symptom compromises or with the inclusion of regressed behavior. From this point of view, many "psychiatric" states may be regarded as the adaptive form or modality most appropriate to the individual in his life course. Stabilization of these states represents an ecological balance, but this we should then not regard as illness, but as a specialized form of social compensation.

The conditions which cause latent or quiescent symptoms to become manifest, or which produce fresh symptoms, are largely social or environmental; they are the happenings which the person experiences as threats to his coping capacities. The social situation in this connection consists of the significant others in a person's life at the particular time. It is the matrix of meaningful personal associations which are directly available to the individual. Distress occurs when the inherent attitude of unquestioned confidence in social belonging, and in the virtue and protectiveness of the group is undermined. The "protective group" in other words consists of the people whom the individual identifies in his implicit thinking as important to him, and whose relationship to himself he defines implicitly in security supply terms.

How a group of this kind may be influential in the development and containment of psychiatric symptoms may best be illustrated by examples from certain kinds of closed or controlled institutions, such as the doctor-patient relationship in psychotherapy, the child-care institution, and the military services. The process of influence is more visible and more readily observed under these relatively artificial conditions than in an open society. The chief reason for this, of course, is that control of the individual is built into the relationship character of these closed social structures. I pick the particular examples because I have had a good deal of direct personal experience with them, and am, therefore, in a position to report my own observations.

An almost routine illustration of symptom recession is seen early in psychotherapy as transference eases distress. Symptoms appear again during periods of difficulty in the working through of problems, and may become urgently persistent, sometimes in the form in which they were originally presented, as termination becomes a subject for consideration. Almost any kind of symptom manifestation is useful coin in a patient to doctor relationship; the patient conveys his estimate of the situation, his complaints about its progress, and his demands of his physician, in the timing, the mode of presentation, and the emotional qualities of symptom displays. Psychotherapy does not deal with symptoms but with their underlying problems, yet symptoms occupy a proud position as "tickets of admission" to treatment, as an important area of professional interest, and as a communicative binding-material by which patients and doctors establish a basis for mutual, communicative rapport. The dyadic relationship in therapy as a unique social experience receives its validation from the shared interest in the ritual of symptom exploration, which in itself is actually of only indirect therapeutic import.

Examples in the military services of the social character of symptom vicissitude are common. One notes that an abrupt change in life circumstances is never easily tolerated, but its consequences may be particularly disturbing in individuals whose coping margin has been at best tenuous and thin, and whose security has been based on a relatively rigid adaptation to an accustomed web of circumstance. These are generally inflexible personalities with an early life history of emotional deprivation, who have developed a high degree of social and personal compliance as a major defense in dealing with their environment. It is not necessarily the abruptness of the change in environment but its character of intolerance of their compliant defenses, which exposes the inadequacy of their coping capacities. A large number of persons with this kind of difficulty could be observed among those with the so-called "weak-back" syndrome in military inductees. They were pleasant and ingratiating, but completely incapacitated by complaints of low-back pain, or inability to maintain an erect position; it was apparent that they could not carry the burden of their new situation.

Successful adaptation in the military service, however, particularly in combat, depended to a considerable extent on group cohesion and solidarity, and these in turn were based on the special character of military training, heavily invested with psychological indoctrination, in which ambivalences to officer leadership were exploited both to defend group integrity and to permit the outward displacement of mobilized aggression and hostility.[7] A combat group develops a shared superego which sanctions the killing of the enemy, and in which leader authority serves to promote group cohesion and in turn symptom control. The democracy of danger also plays an important role in sustaining group identifications.

As a final example, I cite the well-managed child-care institution, which receives acutely disturbed children, and is generally able to provide them in a relatively short time with a sense of place and belonging, in which they feel cared for and protected, in which their individual needs are attended to and respected, and in which they experience a quickening sense of their own worth and of their right to their own expressiveness. Despite generally traumatic backgrounds, a surprisingly large number of the children manage to achieve ego stabilization, and a generally useful adaptive capacity.

Symptom formation and containment may thus be said to be largely dependent upon the individual's ability to achieve a sense of integration with a meaningful group. A primary function of social systems is to provide opportunities for such achievement; in many ways it is, perhaps, the most necessary matrix for a system's functioning and survival, just as it is necessary for the individual's. The emergence of symptoms as acutely felt experiences is a signal of disturbance in the patterning of meaningful group experience.[8] It may be regarded as an index of social disorder. It is not as such a measure of psychopathology, nor does the wide distribution of symptoms in a society indicate that its people are ill, rather that there are dislocations or disintegrations in the protective social fabric, so that the potential for symptom display becomes progressively more manifest.

The relation of symptoms to illness remains an obscure area. Where there is illness, there will always be found symptoms. However, symptoms may be subsumed by the achievement of ecological balance under the general house-keeping functions of the ego in such a way that the individual experiences no sense of distress, or malfunction, or need of care. Depth therapy, which provides the opportunity for intensive study of the intricacies of psychiatric disorder, is in itself not a reliable method for the evaluation of illness, since it cannot be carried out effectively without encouraging the patient's regression in the service of therapy, but in doing so obscures his personality strengths and capacities. Under optimum social conditions, it seems likely that a good deal of psychiatric symptomatology could be reduced to relative un-importance, and a good deal of psychiatric illness could be modified and controlled to a considerable extent, minimizing the intensity and duration of disabling effects.[9] Such opti-mum conditions, however, are more likely to arise out of favorable political and economic developments than as the result of social or psychosocial management of people.

To summarize what has been said: Symptoms are not as such, indicators of disturbance, and should not be looked at solely in the perspective of psychopathology. They are the products of inevitable conflicts and disturbances in the de-velopmental process, and are subsumed within the general integrating structure of the ego. They are subject to many vicissitudes, remaining latent or manifest at different times and under varying circumstances, or becoming transformed into different symptoms or into character traits. They are not generally associated with a sense of illness but are more often regarded in much the same way as other personality manifestations. They may become more prominent under conditions of distress, or their presence may be elicited and their importance overemphasized through psychiatric exam-ination. If not in themselves indicators of illness, they are among the characteristic expressions of the person who becomes ill. This suggests that epidemiological studies based upon the eliciting of symptoms give a grossly exaggerated picture of the prevalence of mental illness.

Examples have been cited which indicate that the morale

of the key groups with which the individual is identified is of importance in determining his ability to deal with his latent psychopathology, with the extent to which psychopathology will develop and tend to maintain itself, and finally to the person's readiness to regard himself and present himself as psychiatrically disturbed. It seems clear that symptoms may be controlled to a considerable extent in "closed" social systems. There is as yet little evidence that such control is possible in an "open" society. On the other hand, it is of interest to observe that forces within the social structure and within the ego system tend to exert consistent pressure toward ecological stabilization and, thereby, the ordering of symptoms to the life interests of the individual.

The Dynamics of the Psychotherapeutic Relationship

JEROME D. FRANK

All forms of psychotherapy, whatever their underlying theories, and whatever techniques they employ, attempt to promote beneficial changes in a patient's attitudes and symp-

FROM *Psychiatry* 22 (Feb., 1959) 17–34. Reprinted by permission of the author and the publisher.

This paper has grown in part out of research studies supported by the United States Public Health Service (M-532, C-2) and the Ford Foundation. Many of the ideas have been developed and clarified through discussion with Lester H. Gliedman, M.D., Stanley D. Imber, Ph.D., Earl H. Nash, Jr., M.S., and Anthony R. Stone, M.S.S.W., members of the Henry Phipps Psychiatric Clinic of the Johns Hopkins Hospital psychotherapy research staff, to whom the writer expresses his appreciation.

toms through the influence of a therapist with whom the patient has a close relationship. The purpose of this paper is to review data from diverse sources bearing on the determinants and effects of the patient's emotional dependency on his psychotherapist for relief. The effects may include modifications of the patient's productions in the interview, the duration of treatment itself, and changes in the patient's attitudes and bodily states. Certain mechanisms which may transmit the therapist's expectancies to the patient will be described, and some implications of these data for research and practice will be briefly considered. The major sources of material are reports concerning brainwashing, miracle cures, experimental studies of the psychotherapeutic interview, and the placebo effect.

In general terms, all psychotherapies are concerned with using the influence of the therapist to help patients to unlearn old, maladaptive response patterns and to learn better ones, but they differ considerably in their specific goals and methods. Examples of goals are helping the patient to recover early memories, develop insight, work through transference relationships, release his spontaneity or modify his self-concept. Methods include, for example, free association, client-centered interviews, and progressive relaxation. These differences in therapeutic approach are reflected in differences in the patient's behavior and in the kinds of change resulting from treatment.

In addition to the differing effects of the psychotherapist's influence which depend on his particular orientation and method, all forms of psychotherapy seem to produce certain similar effects based on a quality common to the relationships they offer. This common feature is the patient's reliance on the therapist to relieve his distress.

This reliance, which may be forced or voluntary, arises from the interplay of environmental pressures and the patient's subjective state, the relative contribution of each differing from case to case. An example of forced reliance produced primarily by environmental pressure would be the situation of a paranoid patient, placed in a hospital against his will, who believes his incarceration to be unjust, but who is nevertheless forced to depend on the staff to gain his release. An example of forced reliance arising from subjective pressure would be the patient in a panic who flees to the psychiatrist for protection. More commonly, especially in office practice, the patient's dependence on the psychiatrist is voluntary and arises from the interplay of more subtle environmental and subjective factors. These lead the patient to expect relief from the psychiatrist, an expectancy which sometimes may be strong enough to justify the term *faith*.

DETERMINANTS OF THE PATIENT'S RELIANCE ON HIS PSYCHOTHERAPIST

Conditions maintaining or strengthening a patient's reliance on his psychotherapist to relieve his suffering may be conveniently grouped under four headings: the culture, the treatment situation, the therapist, and the patient.

The Culture

The beliefs of members of a culture as to what constitutes illness and its treatment are formed and supported by generally held cultural attitudes.[1] A member of a particular society can regard himself as having an emotional illness— for which the proper treatment is psychotherapy—only if his society recognizes the existence of such illnesses and sanctions psychotherapy as the appropriate treatment for them. The same symptoms which in the Middle Ages were viewed as signs of demoniacal possession to be treated by exorcism, are now regarded as manifestations of mental illness to be treated by a psychiatrist. In World War II Russian soldiers did not have psychoneuroses, which can only mean that the Russian army did not recognize the existence of such conditions. Presumably soldiers with functional complaints were regarded either as malingerers, and thus subject to disciplinary action, or as medically ill, and therefore to be treated by regular physicians. In the American army, by contrast, many commonplace reactions to the stresses of military life were initially regarded as signs of psychoneurosis. Soldiers with these complaints, therefore, often received psychotherapy, which not infrequently culminated in their discharge. Today many of these same soldiers would be promptly returned to active duty.

In mid-century America, mental illness has not fully shaken off its demonological heritage, as evidenced by the stigma still attached to it. Both psychotics and neurotics, however, are seen as suffering from bona fide illnesses, and the dominant treatment for most of the conditions subsumed under mental and emotional illness is psychotherapy. Moreover, the psychiatrist is generally regarded as the best qualified dispenser of this form of treatment, although other professional groups are challenging his right to this pre-eminence. Therefore an American today, once he has accepted the label of being mentally or emotionally ill, is culturally predisposed to expect relief from psychotherapy and to look to a psychiatrist for this relief.

The Treatment Situation

Certain situations in which psychotherapy is practiced, notably mental hospitals, to a varying degree force the patient to become dependent on the treatment staff. Even when there is no external compulsion, however, many aspects of the psychotherapeutic situation in both hospital and office supply cues which tend to impress the patient with the importance of the procedure, and also to identify psychotherapy with other healing methods. In both ways they strengthen his expectation of relief and thus his dependency on the therapist. The cues start to operate before the patient and therapist meet. Most patients reach the presence of the psychotherapist only after some preliminaries. If the patient is hospitalized, the commitment procedure heightens his sense of dependence on the hospital staff for his release. Voluntary admission procedures usually require the patient to sign a witnessed request for admission which contains a "three-day notice" clause. This impresses him with the importance of the step he is taking and underlines the staff's control over him while in the hospital. If properly conducted, the admission procedure can heighten the patient's hope of benefit from his stay and his trust in the treatment staff.

Psychiatrists working with outpatients are rightly concerned that the referral heighten the patient's favorable expectations, rather than making him feel that he is being 'brushed off'—a situation which frequently occurs. One of the purposes of the intake procedure of psychiatric outpatient clinics is to predispose the patient favorably to psychotherapy. At the Phipps Clinic, for example, each new patient is first briefly interviewed by a trained nurse as a deliberate reminder that he is under medical auspices.

More commonly, patients coming to a psychiatric clinic first have one or more intake interviews with a social worker. The avowed purposes of these are to determine the patient's suitability for psychotherapy and to prepare him for it. The patient may, however, perceive the intake process as a probationary period to determine his worthiness to receive the psychiatrist's ministrations. Thus subtly impressing him with the importance of psychotherapy heightens his susceptibility to the psychiatrist's influence. In this sense the intake procedure is analogous to the preparatory rites undergone by suppliants at faith healing shrines, with the social worker in the role of acolyte and the psychiatrist as high priest.

Once in the presence of his therapist, the patient's favorable expectancies are reinforced by the setting. Psychotherapy has developed its own trappings, to symbolize healing; like other physicians, psychotherapists display diplomas prominently, but in place of the symbols of the stethoscope, the opthalmoscope, and the reflex hammer, they must rely on the heavily laden bookcases, the couch, the easy chair, and usually a large photograph of the leader of their particular school looking benignly but impressively down on the proceedings. In medical institutions, much of the same effect is created simply by the locale of the psychiatrists' offices, which identifies them with the healing activities of the hospital.[2]

The therapist's activities in the initial interview may also have the function, in part, of heightening the patient's favorable expectancies. Psychiatrists usually take a history, loosely following the model of a medical history, thereby reinforcing their identification with the medical profession in the patient's mind. Psychologists frequently begin by giving the patient a battery of psychological tests, their badge of special competence. Both are apt to conclude the interview by offering the patient some sort of formulation which impresses him with their ability to understand and help him.

In the early days of psychoanalysis, before the setting and procedures had achieved their symbolic power, the analyst might have found it necessary to impress the patient by other means. This is illustrated by Freud's example of the patient who failed to shut the door to the waiting room. He pointed out that this omission

> ... throws light upon the relation of this patient to the physician. He is one of the great number of those who seek authority, who want to be dazzled, intimidated. Perhaps he had inquired by telephone as to what time he had best call, he had prepared himself to come on a crowd of suppliants. . . . He now enters an empty waiting room which is, moreover, most modestly furnished, and he is disappointed. He must demand reparation from the physician for the wasted respect that he has tendered him, and so he omits to close the door between the reception room and the office. . . . He would also be quite unmannerly and supercilious during the consultation if his presumption were not at once restrained by a sharp reminder.[3]

In terms of this discussion, Freud interpreted the patient's behavior as expressing a lack of confidence in him as a successful healer, and sought to restore this confidence by a brusque command.

As treatment progresses, the therapist instructs the patient in certain activities which are based on a particular theory. Whatever their specific nature, all implicitly convey that the therapist knows what is wrong with the patient and that the special procedure is the treatment for it. In addition, the underlying theory supplies a frame of reference which helps the patient to make sense of behavior and feelings which had been mysterious and to learn that they are not unique, but represent important and widely shared experiences.

Thus from the moment the prospective patient approaches psychotherapy until his treatment terminates, he is confronted with cues and procedures which tend to impress him with both the importance of the procedure and its promise of relief. These heighten the therapist's potential influence over the patient and, as will be discussed below, probably have some therapeutic effects in themselves by mobilizing his favorable expectations.

The Therapist

In addition to as yet ill-defined personal characteristics, two attitudes of the therapist foster the patient's confidence in him. One is his faith in the patient's capacity to benefit from treatment, which is implied in the mere act of accepting him as a patient. The therapist's acceptance of the patient may be influenced by his own feelings. In his first publication on psychotherapy Freud wrote:

The procedure . . . presupposes . . . in [the physician] . . . a personal concern for the patients. . . . I cannot imagine bringing myself to delve into the psychical mechanism of a hysteria in anyone who struck me as low-minded and repellent, and who, on closer acquaintance, would not be capable of arousing human sympathy.[4]

Similar considerations make some psychotherapists unwilling to accept alcoholics or patients with antisocial character disorders for treatment. Schaffer and Myers[5] have found that middle-class clinic patients, more often than lower-class ones, are assigned to senior staff members, who presumably have first choice. They relate this to the fact that middle-class patients appear to offer better prospects for therapy because their values are closer to those of the psychiatrists. The therapist's faith in the capacities of his patient is a strong incentive to maintain that attitude of active personal participation which helps the patient to develop confidence in him.[6]

The other therapeutically potent attitude of the therapist is his confidence in his theory and method of treatment. How these enhance the therapeutic meaning of the treatment situation in the patient's eyes has been touched on above. Adherence to a definite therapeutic procedure and theory also helps to maintain the psychotherapist's confidence. As one young analyst remarked, "Even if the patient doesn't improve, you know you're doing the right thing."

In fields where there is a common body of validated knowledge and the effectiveness of treatment has been demonstrated—for example, abdominal surgery or infectious disease—the physician's confidence rests on his mastery of the pertinent knowledge and diagnostic and therapeutic techniques. In psychotherapy, which lacks such a body of information, therapists tend to rely for their emotional security on allegiance to a group which represents a particular view. This allegiance is fostered by a long period of indoctrination, as many writers have pointed out.[7] Glover, who deplores the effect of this on the research capacities of young psychoanalysts, writes:

> It is scarcely to be expected that a student who has spent some years under the artificial . . . conditions of a training analysis and whose professional career depends on overcoming "resistance" to the satisfaction of his training analyst, can be in a favorable position to defend his scientific integrity against his analyst's theories and practice. . . . For according to his analyst the candidate's objections to interpretations rate as "resistances." In short there is a tendency inherent in the training situation to perpetuate error.[8]

The effectiveness of indoctrination in psychotherapy is suggested by replies of a group of psychotherapists—mainly Freudian, Adlerian, or Jungian in orientation—to a questionnaire distributed by Werner Wolff.[9] Seventy percent stated that they believed their particular form of therapy to be the best, a high figure considering the absence of any objective data that one form of therapy is superior to another.[10] Only 25 percent, however, professed themselves satisfied with their theoretical orientation. It is interesting that these consisted mostly of disciples of Adler and Jung. Wolff comments: "The degree of identification of each member with the leader of the group is greater in minority groups, which defend their new system against the system of the majority group."[11] Thus 45 percent, or about half of those who responded, believed their therapy to be best, not only in the absence of objective evidence but also without being sure of the soundness of the theory on which it was based. This is a striking testimonial to the faith of those therapists in their procedures.

It seems safe to conclude that training in psychotherapy tends to develop a strong allegiance in the young therapist to his therapeutic school. This contributes to his confidence in his brand of treatment, which, in turn, helps him to inspire confidence in his patients.

At this point it seems appropriate to mention that the factors so far enumerated which enhance the patient's faith in psychotherapy in the United States are remarkably similar to those reported with respect to shamanism in Indian tribes. Henri Ellenberger, for example, points out that among the Kwakiutl Indians, "to become a shaman requires a four-year program in a kind of professional school with strict rules. The shamans constitute a corporation and possess a considerable body of knowledge which they are anxious to transmit to qualified persons."[12] He mentions four factors to which the success of shamanistic cures is attributed. These are: the faith of the shamans in their own abilities, the faith of the patient in the healer's abilities, the acknowledgement of the disease by the social group, and the acceptance of the healing method by the group. Shamans do not treat all diseases, many of which are treated by natural medications or plants; but there are special diseases for which the intervention of the shaman is the only recourse.

The Patient

The extent to which a patient accepts the cues offered by the culture, the treatment situation, and his therapist as representing potential relief depends, of course, also on his own attributes. Many complex and as yet poorly understood factors influence a patient's ability to develop trust in his therapist. In a recent study of patients in a psychiatric clinic, more of those who remained in individual psychotherapy at least six months than of those who dropped out within the first month were suggestible, as measured by a sway test.[13] This study also confirmed the results of Schaffer and Myers with respect to social and educational status and remaining in treatment.[14] That is, patients whose values were such that the goals and methods of psychotherapy made sense to them were more likely to stay in treatment.

Perhaps the major personal determinant of the patient's faith in treatment is the degree of his distress. The literature is consistent in the finding that with neurotics the degree of reported distress is positively related to remaining in treatment.[15] There are at least two possible, and compatible, explanations of this. One, which is consistent with the little that is known about miracle cures, is that presumably the more wretched a person is, the greater his hunger for relief and the greater his predisposition to put faith in what is offered.[16] The other possibility is that the patient's revelation of distress is in itself a sign that he is favorably disposed to trust the therapist and therapy; that is, it may indicate a willingness on the part of the patient to emphasize aspects of himself which show his vulnerability or weakness.

MODES OF TRANSMISSION OF THE THERAPIST'S INFLUENCE

That the psychotherapist influences his patients is generally accepted. Early psychotherapeutic techniques such as mesmerism, direct suggestion under hypnosis, and the moral persuasion of Dubois deliberately exploited the therapist's power. Directive forms of psychotherapy still dominate the treatment scene in their modern forms of hypnotherapy, progressive relaxation, directive counseling, and simple advice-giving. Of Wolff's respondents, most of whom, it will be remembered, were trained in the broad psychoanalytical tradition, only 27 percent said they used a strictly nondirective approach.[17]

Nevertheless, beginning with Freud's substitution of so-called free association for hypnosis, the dominant trend in writings on psychotherapy has emphasized the desirability of the therapist's using more indirect methods of influence. The goals of treatment are expressed in more ambitious terms than the relief of the patient's distress and improvement of his functioning. He must be helped toward greater self-actualization, spontaneity, maturity, creativity, and the like. The therapist facilitates the patient's movement by empathizing with him, accepting him, collaborating with him, respecting him, and being permissive. The patient's natural tendency to be dependent on the therapist is to be combatted. The therapist is not to persuade or advise, since such activities impede the patient's growth toward emotional maturity.

This trend may spring in part from democratic values, which place a higher worth on apparently self-directed, spontaneous behavior than on that obviously caused by outside influence.[18] The swing from directive techniques also derives in part from the experience that many cures achieved through these means proved to be transitory, although whether a larger percentage of enduring results is achieved by more permissive techniques is still unknown.

I shall now review some ways in which the therapist may transmit his expectancies to the patient and so influence the latter's productions in treatment, often without the awareness of either. Data are adduced from two sources: Chinese thought reform or brainwashing, and content analyses of patients' and therapists' verbalizations in treatment.

Chinese Thought Reform

At first glance, nothing could seem more remote from psychotherapy than methods used by Chinese Communists to obtain confessions from their prisoners. The objects of psychotherapy are patients; those of thought reform, prisoners. Patients and therapists operate within the same broad cultural framework; the cultural values of interrogators and prisoners clash. The goals of psychotherapist and patient are roughly similar; those of interrogator and prisoner are diametrically opposed. In psychotherapy the welfare of the patient is uppermost; in thought reform that of the prisoner is of no account. Thought reform relies on the application of extreme force; psychotherapy typically eschews overt pressure on the patient.

Nevertheless, several psychiatrists have been impressed by certain parallels between psychotherapy and thought reform;[19] in both someone in distress must rely on someone else for relief, and in both the person in distress is required to review and reinterpret his past life in detail. Just as the study of pathological processes increases the understanding of normal ones by throwing certain of their characteristics into relief, a study of thought reform, which may be regarded as a pathological form of psychotherapy, highlights some aspects of the latter which have received inadequate attention.

Thought reform utilizes both group and individual pressures to break down the prisoner's sense of personal identity and influence him to assume a new one incorporating the attitudes and values of his captors. The victim is snatched from his usual activities and abruptly plunged into a completely hostile environment. Present miseries are compounded by threats of worse to come, with the possibility of death always present. Physical tortures are of the humiliating type, such as manacling the prisoner's hands behind his back so that he has to eat like an animal. He receives none of the respect or consideration accorded to his previous status. For example, he is allowed only a few moments to defecate and must do it in public. He is completely immersed in a group which incessantly hammers at his values and demands that he adopt theirs. The group's attitude is implacable and rigidly consistent. For example, the group assumes that the prisoner is guilty and that the enormity of his offenses justifies the harshest punishment. Therefore, any punishment he does receive is a sign of his captor's leniency. The effect of these pressures on the prisoner is strengthened by complete severance of his contact with former associates, and he receives only such distorted and fragmentary news of the outer world as fits the aims of his captors. By these means his sense of personal identity is weakened and his critical faculties are dulled, decreasing his ability to resist.

The prisoner is removed from the group only for the time he spends with an interrogator, whose task it is to obtain the prisoner's "confession" of his "crimes." Certain features of the interrogation situation are relevant to this discussion. It is characterized by rigidity in some respects, by ambiguity in others, by repetition, and by insistence on the prisoner's participation.

The rigidity lies in the interrogator's attitude of infallibility. His position is that the Communist viewpoint on every issue is the only correct one. The prisoner's guilt is axiomatic, and all his productions are judged in the light of this assumption. The interrogator indicates that he knows what the crimes are, but the prisoner must make his own confession. He is encouraged to talk or write freely about himself and his alleged crimes, but he is not told what to write. He may be punished severely, however, if his production does not accord with the desires of his interrogator. Those statements which do meet the interrogator's wishes gain approval, which reinforces them the more effectively because of the prisoner's previous apprehensiveness.[20] No matter what he confesses, it is never enough, but the hope continues to be held out to him that once he makes a proper and complete confession he will be released. The prisoner is thus placed in a perceptually ambiguous situation which compels him to scrutinize the interrogator for clues as to what is really wanted, while at the same time offering him no target against which to focus his resistance.

The participation of the prisoner in bringing about his own change of attitude is implicit in this procedure. By putting the responsibility for writing an adequate confession on him, his captors force him to commit himself to the process. Schein describes the same procedure in Korean prison camps: "It was never enough for the prisoner to listen and absorb; some kind of verbal or written response was always demanded. . . . The Chinese apparently believed that if they could once get a man to participate . . . eventually he would accept the attitudes which the participation expressed.[21]

Finally, repetition is an important component of thought reform: "One of the chief characteristics of the Chinese was their immense patience in whatever they were doing . . . they were always willing to make their demand or assertion over and over again. Many men pointed out that most of the techniques used gained their effectiveness by being used in this repetitive way until the prisoner could no longer sustain his resistance."[22]

Under these pressures the prisoner's self-searchings produce material increasingly in line with the interrogator's desires, and eventually the victim may be unable to tell fact from fantasy. In extreme cases he accepts his fabricated confession as true. Lifton tells of a man who confessed with conviction and in detail that he had tried to attract the attention of an official representative of his country who passed by the door of his cell, only to discover later that the episode could not possibly have occurred.[23]

The world of the victim of thought reform seems a far cry from that of the mental patient, and yet the analogies are sometimes startling. Some patients are in the same state of terror and bewilderment that the Communists try to produce in their prisoners. To quote Hinkle and Wolff,

In all [the Communist indoctrination programs] the subject is faced with pressure upon pressure and discomfort upon discomfort, and none of his attempts to deal with his situation lead to amelioration of his lot. Psychiatrists may refer to a man in such a situation as "emotionally bankrupt." Some of the patients who seek the help of psychiatrists are in a similar state. The pressures and convolutions of their lives have reached a point at which they can no longer deal with them, and they must have help. It is recognized that such a state of "emotional bankruptcy" provides a good opportunity for the therapist.[24]

Furthermore, some interrogators are analogous to psychotherapists in two respects. Their contact with the prisoner is close and prolonged, and they see themselves as trying to promote the prisoner's true welfare by getting him to discard his unhealthy, outmoded values and attitudes and adopt the "healthier" ones of the Communist ideology. Under these conditions it is not surprising that intense transferences and countertransferences can develop between a prisoner and his interrogator.

As Erving Goffman has vividly pointed out, mental hospitals, in the eyes of many patients, may display some of the characteristics of the Communist prisons.[25] Patients are deprived of their usual badges of personal identity and are forced into a humiliating position of complete dependence on the treatment staff for even such small things as cigarettes. They are cut off from their contacts with the outer world and totally immersed in a different culture. They see themselves as completely in the power of the staff, whose decisions often appear to them to be arbitrary or capricious. They know that in order to get out they must satisfy the demands of the staff, but they have no clear idea as to how to do this.

Moreover, the ideology of the mental hospital is consistently and rigidly maintained. Thus all measures applied to the patient, such as transfer from an open to a locked ward, are perceived by the staff as "therapy." If the patient demurs, he is met with what Goffman calls the "institutional smirk," with its implication that "you may think that's what you want, but we know better." Although this somewhat malicious description deliberately highlights the coercive aspects of the mental hospital, the caricature is not so extreme as to be unrecognizable.

The parallels between thought reform and outpatient psychiatry, whether in clinic or private practice, are much fainter, but they can still be discerned. As with hospitalized patients, the psychiatrist's potential influence on the outpatient depends in part on the latter's expectancy of help. A few office patients turn to the psychiatrist as a last resort after having vainly tried other possible sources. Their favorable expectancy, like that of many hospitalized patients, is based on desperation. A larger group are not sure why they have come to the psychiatrist or how the latter can help them. The psychiatrist then has the task of mobilizing their favorable expectancies by convincing them that they are ill, and that the illness is best treated by psychotherapy. This is usually expressed as arousing the patient's consciousness of illness. As Kubie writes: "Without a fullhearted acknowledgment of the sense of illness a patient can go through only the motions of treatment."[26]

Moreover, he writes, "it is often necessary during an analysis to lead a patient through a sustained period of relative isolation from his usual activities and human associations."[27] It may not be entirely farfetched to read into such a statement a recognition that a patient, like the prisoner, can more easily be brought to change his ideology if he is removed from the groups which reinforce his current one.

Viewing psychotherapy in the light of thought reform calls attention to another feature which tends to enhance the therapist's influence. This is his interpretation of all of the patient's thoughts, feelings, and acts in terms of a consistent and unshakable theoretical framework. In accordance with his theory, the therapist assumes that the patient's distress is related to repressed infantile memories, parataxic distortions, or an unrealistic self-image, to take three examples.

Therapy continues until the patient acknowledges these phenomena in himself and deals with them to the therapist's and his own satisfaction. The possibility that he has not experienced the phenomena in question or that they may be irrelevant to his illness is not entertained. Freud's handling of his discovery that patients confabulated infantile memories may serve as a prototype of this way of thinking. As he was quick to see, "this discovery . . . serves either to discredit the analysis which has led to such a result or to discredit the patients upon whose testimony the analysis, as well as the whole understanding of neurosis, is built up." A bleak predicament indeed, from which Freud extricates himself by a tour de force. He points out that "these phantasies possess *psychological* reality in contrast to *physical* reality," and *"in the realm of neuroses the psychological reality is the determining factor."*[28] Therefore the fact that these infantile experiences were fantasies rather than actualities, far from refuting his theories, actually confirms them. The Freudian theory of neurosis rests on more solid evidence than real or fabricated infantile memories, of course. The purpose of this example is to illustrate a type of thinking which is characteristic of psychotherapists and which contributes to their influence on patients.

The therapist may protect the infallibility of his theoretical orientation in subtle ways. For example, behavior of patients which does not conform to his position is apt to be characterized as "resistance," or "manipulation." Patients' criticisms can always be dismissed as based on "transference," implying that they are entirely the result of the patient's distorted perceptions. Faced with such behaviors, the therapist is admonished not to become "defensive"—that is, not to admit, even by implication, that his viewpoint requires defending.

The therapist also has ways of maintaining his faith in his theory and procedures in the face of a patient's failure to respond favorably. He may take refuge in the position that the patient broke off treatment too soon. Or he may conclude that the patient was insufficiently motivated or otherwise not suitable for treatment. Occasionally he may entertain the possibility that he applied his technique incorrectly, but failures rarely lead him to question the technique itself or the premises underlying it. In short, the vicissitudes of treatment are not permitted to shake the therapist's basic ideology.

In calling attention to the means by which psychotherapists maintain their conviction of the correctness of their theories and procedures, I imply no derogation. On the contrary, this conviction probably is partly responsible for the success of all forms of psychotherapy. I stress it here as one of the ingredients which heighten the therapist's influence on the patient.

The methods of psychotherapy, finally, are slightly analogous to those of thought reform with respect to repetition, participation, and ambiguity. In long-term psychotherapy, the patient repeatedly reviews material connected with certain issues, toward which the therapist maintains a consistent attitude. That this may tend to influence the patient in accordance with the therapist's viewpoint is consistent with what is known concerning the role of repetition in all learning.

The desirability of the patient's being an active participant or collaborator in the treatment process is universally recognized. One of the many reasons for encouraging such an attitude is that it forestalls or combats the patient's tendency to become dependent on the therapist. Yet the perspective of thought reform suggests that it may also heighten the therapist's influence in at least two ways. The more the patient's active participation can be obtained, the more he commits himself to the change which the therapist is trying to induce. Moreover, the patient has greater difficulty in mobilizing his resistance against a collaborative than a directive therapist.

It is in the ambiguity of the therapeutic situation, however, that its greatest potentiality for influence probably lies. Like the interrogators in thought reform, some psychotherapists convey to the patient that they know what is wrong with him but that he must find it out for himself in order to be helped. This is one means of enlisting his participation, but it also gives the patient an ambiguous task.[29] This ambiguity is heightened by the fact that the end-point of this process, whether it be unearthing his infantile memories, making his unconscious conscious, correcting his idealized image, or what not, is indeterminate, like that of the confession. The patient is to keep on trying until he is cured, but the criteria which will indicate that cure has been achieved are not clearly specified.

Psychotherapists have always been alert to the possibility of directly imposing their own ideas in the long-term, repetitive relationship of psychotherapy and have advocated certain attitudes to diminish this possibility. One is permissiveness, that is, the therapist leaves the patient free to use the therapeutic situation as he wishes. The perspective of thought reform suggests that, given a patient who expects the therapist to relieve his distress, the latter's permissiveness, by creating an ambiguous situation, may enhance rather than diminish his power to indoctrinate the patient. By failing to take a definite position, the therapist deprives the patient of a target against which to mobilize his opposition. Furthermore, an ambiguous situation tends to create or increase the patient's confusion, which as Cantril suggests, tends to heighten suggestibility.[30] It also makes him more anxious, therefore presumably heightening his motivation to please the therapist.[31] This motivation is enhanced by the fact that the ambiguity is in a context of threat of unfortunate consequences if the patient does not perform the task properly. In thought reform the threat of punishment for failure is direct; in psychotherapy it is indirectly conveyed by the implication that the patient's distress will not be relieved, and perhaps also by subtle hints of the therapist's disapproval or lack of interest when the patient is not "cooperating." That an ambiguous therapeutic situation may intensify the patient's search for subtle hints as to how well he is doing can be testified to by many analysands, who are acutely aware of changes in the analyst's respiration, when he lights his pipe, shifts in his chair, and so on, even when he is out of their sight.

In summary, factors similar to those in thought reform can, in greatly attenuated form, be discerned in psychotherapy, and may in part determine the strength of the psychotherapist's influence. Changes produced by such means range from mere verbal compliance which vanishes with the disappearance of the influencing agent, to genuine internalization of attitudes and values, depending on personal and situational factors still not understood.[32]

Psychotherapy as Operant Conditioning

A mechanism of transmission of influence which seems analogous to operant conditioning[33] occurs in psychotherapy, according to some experimental evidence, and probably also in thought reform. This technique, which produces extremely rapid learning in animals, consists in reinforcing by a prompt reward some spontaneous act—such as a pigeon's pecking at a target or a rat's hitting a lever with his paw. For example, when the rat hits the lever he receives a pellet of food. Analogously, in psychotherapy the patient's spontaneous behavior is his speech, and the therapist reinforces certain verbalizations by cues of approval which may be as subtle as a fleeting change of expression, or as obvious as an elaborate interpretation.

The reinforcing effect of simple signs of interest lies in the fact that, as Jurgen Ruesch says: "The driving force inherent in any form of psychotherapy is related to the patient's experience of pleasure when a message has been acknowledged. Successful communication is gratifying; it brings about a feeling of inclusion and security and leads to constructive action. Disturbed communication is frustrating; it brings about a feeling of loneliness and despair and leads to destructive action."[34]

The first experimental support of the hypothesis that verbal behavior might be subject to operant conditioning was offered by Greenspoon.[35] He had graduate students say as many words as they could in 50 minutes. He sat behind the subjects and exerted no ostensible control over them. In accordance with a preconceived plan, however, he sometimes said, "Mm-hm," and sometimes, "Huh-uh," just after the subjects used a plural noun. He also introduced other variations as controls. By statistical analysis he showed that "Mm-hm" significantly increased the number of plural nouns spoken by the subjects and "Huh-uh" significantly decreased them.

These effects occurred without the subjects' knowledge that they were being influenced.

Following this lead, experimenters have begun to study the patient's productions in psychotherapy as influenced by the therapist's behavior. Only a few results have been published to date, but they confirm Greenspoon's findings. Salzinger and Pisoni used as subjects 14 female and 6 male schizophrenics newly admitted to the New York State Psychiatric Institute.[36] Each patient was interviewed for 30 minutes, once by a man and once by a woman, on two consecutive days, within one week after arrival. In each interview, for the first ten minutes the interviewer offered no reinforcement. During the next ten minutes he systematically reinforced affect statements by the patient, by simple grunts, looks of interest, and so on. During the third ten minutes, no reinforcement was offered. Affect statements were those defined as those beginning with "I" or "we," followed by an expression of feeling. They found that, with both interviewers, even a ten-minute period of reinforcement significantly increased the frequency of affect statements over both the control periods. Apparently patients learn as fast as pigeons. Murray reports a content analysis of two case protocols, one of his own and one of "Herbert Bryan" published by Rogers.[37] In his patient, "defensive statements" as defined by him, and which he disapproved, fell from 140 to 9 per interview, over 17 sessions. Expressions of hostility, which he permitted—and perhaps subtly reinforced—rose from practically none to nearly 80 by the fourth interview. In Herbert Bryan's protocol, statements in categories disapproved by the therapist fell from 45 percent of the total number of statements in the second hour to 5 percent in the eighth. Statements in approved categories rose from 1 percent in the second hour to 45 percent in the seventh.

The case of Herbert Bryan has particular interest because it was offered as an example of nondirective therapy. The therapist presumably believed that he was not influencing the patient's productions, yet different raters were able to classify his interventions as implicitly approving or disapproving with a high degree of reliability. Apparently a therapist can strongly affect his patient's productions without being aware that he is doing so.

Perhaps other conventional psychotherapeutic maneuvers may also function as positive or negative stimuli for operant conditioning, thereby influencing the patient's productions in the direction of the therapist's expectancies. Silence, for example, when used to indicate lack of interest, might be a negative reinforcer, influencing the patient to desist from those verbalizations which elicit it.

An interpretation can be viewed as having both positive and negative reinforcing potential. It acts as a positive reinforcer by implicitly conveying the therapist's interest in the patient's verbalization, and, more specifically, by heightening its significance. This it does by relating the patient's statement to a larger system of thought, often with dramatic overtones, as is implied by such concepts as, for example, Oedipus complex, persona and anima, and self-actualization. On the negative side, an interpretation of a patient's behavior as resistance—for example, as an implicit indication of the therapist's disapproval—would probably act as a negative reinforcer.

Beyond their function as positive and negative reinforcers, interpretations are the means whereby the therapist presents his self-consistent and unshakable value system to the patient and demonstrates his mastery of a body of theory and technique. In these ways they further contribute to the therapist's influence.

The possibility that interpretations might directly influence the patient's productions has long been recognized. Psychoanalysts in particular have sought to deny that interpretations can operate as suggestion in this sense.[38] The material just cited as well as evidence from psychoanalysis itself casts considerable doubt on this contention. Freud's well-known statement that ". . . we are not in a position to force anything on the patient about the things of which he is ostensibly ignorant or to influence the products of the analysis by arousing an expectation," was made before his discovery that patients fabricated infantile memories in accord with his theories.[39] Glover went to some lengths to draw a distinction between correct and incorrect interpretations, agreeing that the latter might operate by suggestion but offering elaborate reasons why the former did not. That he did not entirely convince himself is suggested by the following quotation, from an article written some twenty years later: ". . . despite all dogmatic and puristic assertions to the contrary we cannot exclude or have not yet excluded the transference effect of 'suggestion through interpretation.' "[40] Recently Carl Rogers has agreed that even his "client-centered" techniques "institute certain attitudinal conditions, and the client has relatively little voice in the establishment of these conditions. We predict that if these conditions are instituted, certain behavioral consequences will ensue in the client. Up to this point this is largely external control."[41]

Operant conditioning offers a mechanism for explaining the repeated observation that patients tend to express their problems and attitudes in the therapist's language. Stekel said long ago, "Dreams are 'made to order,' are produced in the form that will best please the analyst."[42] Patients treated by Carl Rogers' group show a shift of their perceived self toward their ideal self.[43] Those treated by Murray, who operates in a framework of learning theory, show a decrease in defensive verbalizations and an increase in direct expression of feeling.[44] Patients in psychoanalysis express increasing amounts of hitherto unconscious material as treatment progresses. Heine found that veterans who had undergone psychotherapy expressed the reasons for their improvements in terms of the theoretical systems of their therapists.[45] Rosenthal found that improved patients showed a shift in their value systems to those held by the therapist.[46]

It may be tentatively concluded that the elimination of suggestion in the crude sense of directly implanting ideas in the patient does not exclude reinforcement which may influence his productions in the directions expected or desired by the therapist. It would be a mistake, however, to generalize too hastily from these scanty findings. They apply only to what the patient says, not to how he actually feels. In psychotherapy as in thought reform, the extent to which changes in verbalizations represent mere compliance or internalization of the attitudes expressed is unknown.[47] There is a distinct possibility, however, that a person's attitudes may be significantly influenced by his own words. Most persons cannot indefinitely tolerate a discrepancy between communicative behavior and underlying attitudes because such deceit is incompatible with self-respect, and under some conditions it is the attitudes which yield.[48]

The chief interest of operant conditioning for psychotherapy at this point is that it can work through cues of which the therapist is unaware, as in the case of Herbert Bryan. This may lead the therapist erroneously to assume that the patient's productions reflect actual attitudes or experiences, thereby independently verifying his theories, whereas in fact they are responses to his expectancies.

In operant conditioning no learning occurs unless the reinforcement satisfies a need of the animal's. A hungry pigeon will quickly learn to peck at a target if his pecks release pellets of food, but a satiated one will not. By analogy it seems likely that certain behaviors of a person will be conditioned only if they are followed by a reinforcement which meets some motivation in him. Greenspoon's graduate students probably were trying to please him by being good experimental subjects. In this connection Verplanck found that students had only "indifferent" success in trying to condition each other. The successful students seemed to have prestige, suggesting that the procedure succeeded if the subject "cared" about the experimenter's behavior.[49] Apparently very slight motivation may suffice if the subject has no objection to learning the new behavior.

When a person does object to the behavior to which others desire to condition him, presumably the strength of his motive to learn the new behavior would have to be sufficient to outweigh the strength of his resistance. Prisoners undergoing thought reform usually had to be made to feel that pleasing the interrogator offered the only hope of escape from an intolerable situation before they responded to his pressures. Psychiatric patients, like political prisoners, are usually committed to a certain view of the world. Sometimes this view may accord with the therapist's, but this could not account for the fact that therapists of all schools obtain confirmatory material from their patients. In some cases, at any rate, the therapist's viewpoint must conflict with the patient's initial one. The apparent ease with which such patients learn to make statements in line with the therapist's expectancies suggests that they are strongly motivated to win his approval. The most likely source of this motivation would appear to be their expectation that he will relieve their distress.

DIRECT EFFECTS OF FAVORABLE EXPECTATION ON THE DURATION AND OUTCOME OF PSYCHOTHERAPY

Any discussion of the effects of psychotherapy involves the thorny issue of how to define and evaluate improvement. Until general agreement is reached on the criteria of improvement and adequate follow-up data are available, many crucial questions cannot be answered. These include, for example, whether the changes brought about by different forms of psychotherapy are the same or different and whether some types of change are more permanent or basic than others. Under the circumstances I believe that progress can best be made by confining the term *improvement* only to explicitly reported or demonstrable favorable changes in a patient's objective or subjective state. This view regards other commonly used criteria of improvement—for example, greater maturity or personality reorganization—as inferences about the causes of the observed behavioral and subjective changes, or ways of summarizing a group of these changes.[50] In this section, various criteria of improvement are used, depending on the material being reviewed. These are disappearance of a bodily lesion such as a wart or a peptic ulcer, beneficial change in a person's attitudes and life pattern as in religious conversions, and changes in certain experimental measures such as a symptom check list or a self-ideal Q sort.[51] The meager evidence available on the duration of such changes will be presented. No attempt is made to evaluate them in terms of "depth" or "extent," and the reader is left free to draw these inferences for himself.

The Temporal Course of Treatment

That the therapist's expectancies, transmitted to the patient, affect the amount of treatment in relation to improvement is suggested by Clara Thompson's observation that frequency of sessions, over a fairly wide range, seems not to affect either the duration or outcome of therapy. She points out that American psychoanalysts, possibly because they liked long weekends, soon dropped the frequency of sessions from six to five per week. Later, under increasing pressure from the hordes of patients seeking treatment, they reduced the frequency to three times, or even once a week. She states that effective psychoanalysis can be done, in rare cases, even at the latter rate. Moreover, "in actual duration of treatment, in terms of months and years, the patient going five times a week takes about as long to be cured as the patient going three times."[52] She concludes that the passage of time required for the patient to consolidate new insights and incorporate them into his daily living is the crucial variable, rather than amount of therapeutic contact. In view of the previous discussion, an alternative conclusion might be that some therapists have changed their expectancies as to the frequency of visits necessary to relieve their patients but not as to the total duration of treatment required. The patients have obliged by taking as long to get well but not needing to be seen as often.

This leads to consideration of some evidence that the speed of the patient's improvement may be influenced by his understanding of how long treatment will last. There has been a tendency for psychotherapy to become increasingly prolonged when there are no external obstacles to its continuance. Psychoanalyses now often last five or six years. At the Counselling Center of the University of Chicago the average number of sessions increased from 6 in 1949 to 31 in 1954.[53]

This development may be a manifestation of the therapist's need to maintain confidence in his form of treatment and thereby the patient's confidence in him. Rather than admit defeat he keeps on trying until he, the patient, or both are exhausted, or until treatment is interrupted by external circumstances, leaving open the possibility that it might have been successful if the patient could have continued longer. In any case, length of treatment probably reflects in part the therapist's and patient's expectancies. Those who practice long-term psychotherapy find that their patients take a long time to respond; those who believe that good results can be produced in a few weeks claim to obtain them in this period of time.[54] There is no evidence that a larger proportion of patients in long-term treatment improve, or that the improvements are more permanent than in patients treated more briefly. On the other hand, there is some experimental evidence that patients respond more promptly when they know in advance that therapy is time-limited.

Particularly interesting in this regard are two papers on the group treatment of peptic ulcer patients. Fortin and Abse treated nine college students with peptic ulcer, demonstrated by X-ray, with an analytic type of group therapy for one and one-half hours twice a week for about a year. The patients simultaneously received medical treatment for relief of discomfort. In these groups "discussion of ulcer symptomatology was ignored and attention became focussed on basic personality problems."[55] Most of the patients had a flare-up of symptoms during the first month, and three required bed rest in the infirmary. However, during the later part of group psychotherapy—presumably after several months—in addition to favorable personality changes the ulcer symptoms lessened in intensity and frequency. Fortin and Abse state that at the end of the year, "Among the four members who were diagnosed initially prior to group therapy, no recurrence was reported; among the remaining six members with chronic peptic ulcers, where the expected rate of recurrence is over 75 percent for a period of three years' observation, only one student reported a hemorrhage."[56]

Chappell, Stefano, Rogerson, and Pike treated 32 patients with demonstrated peptic ulcers, which had been refractory to medical treatment, by a six-week course of daily didactic group therapy sessions in addition to medical treatment, and compared the results with a matched control group receiving medical treatment only.[57] The therapy group stressed ways of promoting "visceral rest." They report that all but one of the experimental subjects became symptom-free within three

weeks, the period during which Fortin's patients were suffering exacerbations. At the end of three months all but two
were symptom-free.[58] In contrast, 18 of the control group of
20, after an initial good response to the medical regimen,
had had full recurrences of symptoms within this period.
At the end of three years, 28 of the experimental group were
re-examined, and 24 "considered themselves to be healthy."
Of these 15 were symptom-free or nearly so. Only two were
as sick as at the start. Thus Chappell's patients began to get
better while Fortin's were getting sicker, and the end results
seem equally good and at least equally durable.[59]

That patients' expectations concerning the duration of
treatment affect the speed of their response is suggested by
a finding of a research study on psychotherapy of psychiatric
outpatients.[60] Patients were assigned at random to three
psychiatric residents for individual therapy at least one hour
a week, group therapy one and one-half hours a week, or
"minimal individual therapy," not more than one-half hour
every two weeks. Each resident conducted all three types of
treatment. The residents' obligation extended only to six
months of treatment, at which time they were free to drop
the patients. The patients were told that at the end of six
months a decision as to further treatment would be made by
patient and therapist. Two scales were used to measure
patients' progress. One was a symptom check list filled out
by the patient as a measure of his subjective state. The other
was a social ineffectiveness scale, a measure of the adequacy
of social functioning, filled out by the research staff on the
basis of interviews with both the patient and an informant.
At the first re-evaluation, at the end of six months, there was
a sharp average decline in both symptoms and social ineffectiveness. The decline in symptoms was unrelated to type of
therapy or therapist; improvement in social effectiveness was
greater, the greater the amount of treatment contact over
the six-month period. Although individual variations were
marked, discomfort scores and ineffectiveness scores at the
end of two years were on the average no higher than they
were at the end of six months, regardless of whether or not
patients continued in psychotherapy. This raises the possibility that many of these patients achieved their improvement

in six months because they understood this to be the designated period of treatment.

Support for this is offered by Schlien. In a preliminary study which is being checked at this writing, he compared the improvement on certain measures of a group of clients who were told at the start that they would receive only 20 therapeutic sessions over a ten-week period with a group who continued in treatment until voluntary termination. Both groups received client-centered therapy, and the same improvement measures were used for both. The groups were closely matched at the start of therapy by the criteria used. The group receiving time-limited therapy reached the same average level of improvement on these measures at 20 interviews as the others did in 55. Moreover, at the end of the latter period, the group receiving time-limited therapy had maintained their improvement, even though they had been out of treatment several months.[61]

These studies all suggest that speed of improvement may often be largely determined by the patient's expectancies, as conveyed to him by the therapist, as to the duration of treatment, and that a favorable response to brief therapy may be enduring.

Faith as a Healing Agent

For a patient to rely on his therapist for help, he must at least have hope that something useful will transpire. The therapist usually tries to inspire more than this; he seeks to win the patient's trust, confidence, or faith. Many therapists feel that in the absence of such an attitude little can be accomplished; and there is some evidence that this state of mind in itself can have important therapeutic effects.

It is generally agreed that a patient's hope for a successful outcome of treatment can make him feel better, but it is usually assumed that improvement based solely on this is transient and superficial. An example of this type of response is afforded by an obsessional patient who tried several forms of psychotherapy, each lasting many months. He stated that as long as he hoped that the treatment would help him, his symptoms greatly improved. When his hope eventually waned, his symptoms would recur and he would seek another therapist.

Changes following brief therapeutic contact, however, in which little seems to have occurred beyond the arousal of the patient's faith in the therapist, are sometimes deep-seated and persistent. The most plausible explanation for the permanence of these "transference cures" is that the relief the patient experiences from this relationship frees him to function more effectively.[62] He becomes better able to utilize his latent assets and find the courage to re-examine himself and perhaps to modify his habitual maladaptive ways of responding, leading to genuine personality growth.

There is a good possibility, however, that the emotional state of trust or faith in itself can sometimes produce far-reaching and permanent changes in attitude or bodily states, although the occurrence of this phenomenon cannot be predicted or controlled. The major evidence for this lies in the realm of religious conversions and miracle cures.

It is common knowledge that faith in its religious form can have profound and lasting effects on personality, attitudes, and values. After a conversion experience the convert may have changed so much as to be scarcely recognizable as the person he was before this experience. This is seen not only in persons like St. Augustine and St. Francis but even in an occasional denizen of skid row who becomes "saved" at a Salvation Army meeting.[63] Most such conversions are transient, of course, and backsliding is the rule. In this they resemble the transference cures already discussed. As with such cures, perhaps a conversion sticks when it leads to new forms of behavior which yield more rewards than the old patterns. For purposes of this discussion, the only important points are that religious conversions can lead to profound and permanent changes of attitude in persons who have undergone prolonged hardship or spiritual torment and that they usually involve intimate, emotionally charged contact with a person or group representing the viewpoint to which the convert becomes converted. Conversions which occur in isolation are often, perhaps always, preceded by such contacts.[64] According to William James, "General Booth, the founder of the Salvation Army, considers that the first vital step in saving outcasts consists in making them feel that some decent human cares enough for them to take an interest in the question whether they are to rise or sink."[65] The role of divine intervention in producing conversion experiences may be left open. The significant point for this discussion is that they are usually accompanied or preceded by a certain type of relationship with other human beings, which in some ways resembles the psychotherapeutic one. The psychotherapist, too, cares deeply whether his patient rises or sinks.

That faith can also produce extensive and enduring organic changes is amply attested to by so-called miracle cures. There can be little doubt that these cures can activate reparative forces which, in rare instances, are powerful enough to heal grossly damaged tissue. The best documented cases are those healed at Lourdes, and evidence for these is as good as for any phenomena that are accepted as facts.[66]

Patients claiming to have been miraculously cured at Lourdes are examined by a bureau of non-Catholic physicians, who certify that a cure has occurred only when there is unquestioned evidence of organic pathology previous to the cure. The cures include healings of chronic draining fecal fistulas, union of compound fractures which had remained unhealed for years, and similar quite convincing manifestations. Although the consciousness of being cured comes instantly and healing is rapid, it occurs by normal reparative processes. A cachectic patient takes months to regain his weight. An extensive gap in tissues is filled by scar tissue as in normal healing, and this repair may take hours or days.

For various reasons the actual number of cures of this type at Lourdes cannot be accurately calculated. The most conservative figure is the number of cures certified by the Church as miraculous, which by 1955 was only 51. This is an infinitesimal percentage of the millions of pilgrims who visited Lourdes up to that time. By the most liberal criteria, only a small fraction of one percent of the pilgrims have been healed. This raises the possibility that similar cures occur with at least equal frequency in ordinary medical practice but are overlooked because no one physician has a large enough sample of patients. Questioning of colleagues, many of whom report having actually treated or at least having heard of one such case, tends to bear out this supposition. In any case, it is clear that faith cures occur, regardless of the object of the patient's faith. All religions report them, and they are also produced by persons who, by the accepted standards of society, are charlatans. That is, the healing force appears to reside in the patient's state of faith or hope, not in its object. This point has been neatly illustrated by an experiment performed by Rehder with three chronically and severely ill bedridden elderly women patients.[67] One had chronic inflammation of the gall bladder with stones, another had failed to recuperate from an operation for pancreatitis and was a mere skeleton, and the third was in the last stages of metastatic uterine carcinoma. He permitted a local faith healer to try to cure them by absent treatment, without the patients' knowledge. Nothing happened. He next told the patients about the faith healer, built up their expectancies over several days, and then assured them that the faith healer would be treating them from a distance at a certain time the next day. This was a time during which the faith healer did *not* operate. All three women showed dramatic and remarkable improvement at the suggested time. The second was permanently cured; the other two were not, but showed striking temporary responses. The cancer patient, for example, lost massive edema and ascites, her anemia markedly improved, she became strong enough to go home and be up and about, and she continued virtually symptom-free until her death. These three patients were greatly helped by a belief which was false—that the faith healer was treating them from a distance.

Certain features are common to most miracle cures. The patients are usually chronically ill, debilitated, and despondent. Their critical faculty has been weakened, and they are ready to grasp at straws. The journey to the shrine is long and arduous—persons who live in the vicinity of the shrine having proved poor candidates for cures. After arrival there are many preliminaries before the patient can enter the shrine, and during the preparatory period the patient hears about other miraculous cures and views the votive offerings of those healed. As Janet says, "all these things happen today at Lourdes just as they used to happen of old at the temple of Aesculapius."[68] In his despair the patient's state of mind is similar to that of the victim of thought reform, and the symbols of cure are present, as in the psychiatrist's office, although in much more potent form. Finally, all three types of experience are similar in that another person or group of persons is involved who represents the promise of relief.

Since it is the state of hope, belief, or faith which produces the beneficial effects rather than its object, one would expect to find the same phenomena in a nonreligious framework, and this is indeed the case. For example, according to Harold Wolff, hope had definite survival value for prisoners in concentration camps: ". . . prolonged circumstances which are perceived as dangerous, as lonely, as hopeless, may drain a man of hope and of his health; but he is capable of enduring incredible burdens and taking cruel punishment when he has self-esteem, hope, purpose, and belief in his fellows."[69]

In the realm of medicine evidence abounds that faith can facilitate bodily healing. In these cases the patient's faith is activated by the doctor's administration of an inert pharmacological substance, which symbolizes his healing function. Such remedies are called placebos, implying that they are means of placating the patient and therefore not genuine treatment. But placebos can have deep and enduring effects.[70] An instructive example of the power of the placebo is the lowly wart. Warts have been shown by several dermatologists to respond to suggestion as well as to any other form of treatment. One of the most careful studies is that of Bloch.[71] He was able to follow 136 cases of common warts and 43 cases of flat warts over a period of two and one-half years. Of the former group 44 percent, of the latter 88 percent were healed by painting them with an inert dye. About half of the cures occurred after one treatment, while less than 3 percent required more than three sessions. Bloch found that cases which had previously been treated unsuccessfully by the usual means responded just as well as untreated cases, and he adequately ruled out the possibility that his cure rates might represent the percentage that would have healed without any treatment. Since warts are a definite tissue change caused by an identifiable virus, this cure by placebo may serve as a prototype of an organic disease cured by faith.

In this case the faith seems to operate to change the physiology of the skin so that the virus can no longer thrive on it.

Placebos can also heal more serious tissue damage, if it is directly related to the patient's emotional state. In a recently reported study two groups of patients with bleeding peptic ulcer in a municipal hospital in Budapest were compared.[72] The placebo group received an injection of sterile water from the doctor, who told them it was a new medicine which would produce relief. The control group received the same injection from nurses who told them it was an experimental medicine of undetermined effectiveness. The placebo group had remissions which were "excellent in 70 percent of the cases lasting over a period of one year." The control group showed only a 25 percent remission rate. The cure of warts and peptic ulcers by suggestion is not as spectacular as religious miracle cures, but qualitatively the processes involved seem very similar.

Just as placebos can benefit organic conditions, they can help subjective complaints, and the beneficial effects are not necessarily transient. Evidence to support this contention is still scanty. One scrap is that in a controlled study of the effects of mephenesin and placebo on psychiatric outpatients, it was found that the relief of symptoms by placebo persisted undiminished for at least eight weeks, at which time the experiment was terminated.[73]

Miracle cures and placebo responses suggest the probability that a patient's expectancy of benefit from treatment in itself may have enduring and profound effects on his physical and mental state. It seems plausible, furthermore, that the successful effects of all forms of psychotherapy depend in part on their ability to foster such attitudes in the patient. Since it is the patient's state which counts rather than what he believes in, it is not surprising that all types of psychotherapy obtain roughly equal improvement rates.[74] This finding also suggests that the generic type of relationship offered by the therapist plays a larger part in his success than the specific technique he uses. The aspects of the therapist's personality that affect his healing power have not yet been adequately defined, but it seems reasonable to assume that they lie in the realm of his ability to inspire confidence in his patients. In this connection the findings of Whitehorn and

Betz[75] may be pertinent—that therapists whose relationship with their schizophrenic patients was characterized by active personal participation obtained very much better results than those who failed to show this attitude. The therapeutic forces in such a relationship are complex, but one may well be that the therapist's attitude conveys his belief in the patient's capacity to improve, which in turn would strengthen the patient's faith in the treatment procedure, as mentioned earlier. That psychotherapy produces its effects partly through faith is also suggested by the fact that sometimes these effects occur rapidly, as already discussed, and that the speed of cure need bear no relation to its depth or permanence.

The hypothesis that some of the favorable results of psychotherapy may be primarily produced by the patients' favorable expectancies has led some colleagues and myself to study similarities between the effects of psychotherapy and placebo, with the eventual aim of being able to sort out those effects of psychotherapy which cannot be explained on this basis.[76] Two preliminary findings are of interest in this connection. A subgroup of the psychiatric outpatients who were symptomatically improved after six months of psychotherapy, but whose scores on the symptom check list had gradually climbed back to close to the pretreatment level over a two-year follow-up, were then given placebos. After two weeks, their average score on the symptom check list had again dropped back to the level of the period immediately after psychotherapy.[77] The finding that psychotherapy and placebos have similar effects on this measure has led to questions about the meanings of a patient's report of symptoms, which are now being explored. The other tentative finding which has suggested further lines of research is that a group of patients who improved the most on discomfort and ineffectiveness after six months of psychotherapy had personal characteristics surprisingly similar to those found by other investigators in surgical patients whose pain was alleviated by placebos.[78]

In pulling together the evidence that the patient's attitude of trust or faith may play a significant part in his response to all forms of psychotherapy, I do not contend that all or even most of the processes or effects of psychotherapy can be explained on this basis alone. There are obviously many important determinants of the processes and outcomes of treatment besides the direct influence of the therapist based on patients' trust in him. In this presentation, however, I have attempted to focus on two interrelated themes. One is that because of certain properties of all therapeutic relationships, the therapist inevitably exerts a strong influence on the patient. This influence arises primarily from the patient's hope or faith that treatment will relieve his distress. This favorable expectation is strengthened by cultural factors, aspects of the referral or intake process, cues in the therapy situation which indicate that help will be forthcoming, and the therapist's own confidence in his ability to help, springing from his training and his methods. Analogies between psychotherapy and thought reform have been used to clarify some of the sources and modes of operation of the influencing process in the former. Some examples of the influence of the therapist's expectations on the patient's productions and on the duration of therapy have been given.

The other theme is that the patient's favorable expectation, which is a major determinant of the therapist's influence over him, may have direct therapeutic effects which are not necessarily transient or superficial. Certain implications of these propositions for practice and research may be briefly mentioned.

Since this review points out areas of relative ignorance which need further exploration rather than areas of knowledge, its implication for psychotherapeutic practice must be regarded as extremely tentative. It should be noted first that the likelihood of a common factor in the effectiveness of all forms of psychotherapy does not imply that all methods or theories are interchangeable. It may well turn out that the specific effects of different approaches differ significantly and that different types of patients respond differentially to different therapeutic techniques. Until these questions are clarified, it is important that every therapist be well versed in his theoretical orientation and skilled in the methods most congenial to him, in order to maintain his self-confidence and thereby the patient's faith in him. Since the leading conceptual systems of psychotherapy are not logically incompatible, but represent primarily differences in emphasis or alternative formulations of the same ideas,[79] adherents of each school need feel no compunction about holding to their own positions, while tolerant of alternative views, pending the accumulation of facts which may make possible decisions as to the specific merits and drawbacks of different approaches.

If the common effective factor in all forms of psychotherapy is the patient's favorable expectancy, this suggests that psychotherapists should deliberately mobilize and utilize patients' faith in the treatment they offer. The problem here is where to draw the line. The psychotherapist obviously cannot use methods in which he himself does not believe. Moreover, reliance on the healing potentialities of faith to the neglect of proper diagnostic procedures would obviously be irresponsible. Treating tuberculosis or cancer by faith healing alone is none the less reprehensible because it may work occasionally. But a large component of the illnesses which bring patients to psychiatrists—how large is still unclear—consists of harmful emotional states such as anxiety, apprehensiveness, and depression, and for these faith or trust may be a specific antidote. In such conditions, the strengthening of the patient's trust in his therapist, by whatever means, may be as much an etiological remedy as penicillin for pneumonia.

The psychotherapist should be prepared, therefore, to modify his approach, within limits possible for him, to meet the expectancies of different types of patients. Interview types of therapy, for example, tend to fit the expectations of most middle-class patients, but many lower-class patients cannot conceive of a doctor who does not dispense pills or jab them with needles. These patients are very apt to drop out of interview psychotherapy because they cannot perceive it as treatment for their ills.[80] For them the tactics of therapy may involve accommodating to their initial expectations so that they will return for more treatment. The developing therapeutic relationship may then lead to modification of the patients' expectancies in a more psychotherapeutically useful direction. Thus it may be hoped that adequate diagnosis will eventually include an estimate as to the type of therapeutic approach most likely to mobilize the patient's faith.

This review also suggests the desirability that psychotherapists be more aware of the extent of their influence on patients. The physician cannot avoid influencing his patients —the only question is whether he should use this influence consciously or unconsciously.[81] As Modell says, "It would be well to remember that in all therapy trouble is apt to follow the ignorant application of important forces,"[82] and this applies particularly when the important force is the therapist himself.

It might be objected that the therapist's direct use of influence tends to intensify the patient's dependency and thereby impede genuine progress. There is no question as to the desirability of helping patients to independence, but the real problem is to determine when this goal is better achieved by freely accepting their initial dependency and using it, and when by resisting this attitude from the start.[83] It is easy for patient and physician to become absorbed in a struggle over this issue, to the detriment of therapeutic movement. For example, sometimes giving a patient a symptomatic remedy he requests may improve the therapeutic relationship and permit discussion to move to more fruitful topics, whereas withholding it impedes all progress.[84] In order to become genuinely self-reliant, a child needs to feel securely dependent on his parents. From this he develops the confidence in the dependability of others which enables him to forge ahead. The same consideration may often apply to patients.

Validation of these tentative implications for practice awaits the accumulation of more knowledge. This review suggests two hopeful directions in which to seek this knowledge. One is the study of conditions contributing to the patient's faith in his therapist, and the effects of this on the processes and effects of treatment. Psychiatry, in its preoccupation with illness, has concerned itself almost exclusively with pathogenic feelings such as fear, anxiety, and anger. It is high time that the "healing" emotions such as faith, hope, eagerness, and joy received more attention.[85] Of these, the physician-patient relationship affords a special opportunity to study the group of emotions related to expectancy of help which may be grouped under the generic term *faith*. A promising experimental approach to elucidating the determinants, psychological and physiological concomitants, and effects of these emotions lies in study of the placebo effect, since the placebo, under proper circumstances, symbolizes the physician's healing powers. Study of the relationships between the placebo response and response to psychotherapy in psychiatric patients may help to isolate and define the role of the faith component in therapy.

The second promising line of research lies in experimental studies of the ways in which the therapist transmits his expectancies, goals, and values to the patient, and the effects of these on the patient's responses in therapy. Until this matter is elucidated, great caution is advisable in drawing conclusions as to the etiology of mental illness from patients' productions in therapy.

It is now clear that psychotherapists of different schools may elicit from their patients verbal productions confirming the theoretical conceptions of that school and that patients sometimes accommodate their memories and dreams to the expectations of the therapist to the point of outright confabulation. The possibility that the patient may be responding to the therapist's cues and telling him what he wants to hear must always be kept in mind, especially since it can occur without either being aware of it. Hypotheses about interpersonal factors in mental illness require validation by observations outside the therapeutic situation.[86]

By the same token, one must be cautious about attributing improvement to other causes until more is known about the limits of the direct effects of the patient's positive expectancies on his state of health, and the expectancies of the psychiatrist as related to them. Until more is known about the factors in the patient, therapist, and treatment situation which determine the degree and form of influence exerted by the therapist, and about the effects of this influence on the patient's behavior and the nature and duration of his improvement, it is impossible adequately to isolate either the factors specific to each form of psychotherapy or those involved in all forms of psychotherapy. In the meantime there is a danger of falling into the trap of attributing the patient's improvement to the particular kinds of productions he gives in a given kind of treatment, overlooking the possibility that both the productions and the improvement may be determined, at least in part, by his faith in the therapist.

The Obligation to Remain Sick

BEN BURSTEN AND ROSE D'ESOPO

As the scope of psychiatry has broadened, the psychiatric consultant has been requested by his colleagues in internal medicine and surgery to offer assistance with an increasing variety of problems. Prominent among these is management of "difficult" and "uncooperative" patients on medical and surgical wards, and psychiatrists have increasingly become aware that these patients may be responding not only to their individual psychopathology but also to the milieu within which they find themselves. It is the purpose of this paper to discuss and illustrate one aspect of the patient's milieu which may contribute to his illness behavior, and which may lead to the request for psychiatric assistance. This feature of the patient's environment shall be called "the obligation to remain sick."

The focus for this discussion derives from the concept of the sick role which has been defined by Parsons. He has pointed out that "being sick" constitutes a role in society for which there are a set of institutionalized expectations. "Being sick" in this sense, then, is broader than the mere existence

FROM Archives of General Psychiatry 12 (April, 1965) 402–407. Reprinted by permission of the authors and the publisher.

of organic pathology; indeed, many people with organic pathology do not assume the sick role, while others with no discernible change in their organic condition readily assume this role.

Parsons has defined "four aspects of the institutionalized expectations relative to the sick role." Two of these are exemptions: The patient is exempted from his normal social role responsibilities such as supporting his family or participating in activities which might be expected to prolong his illness. The patient is also exempted from a sense of personal responsibility—that is, he is not expected to "pull himself together" nor is he blamed for "acting sick" because he "is sick." There are also two obligations which society defines for the patient. The patient is obliged to want and to try to get well and is further obliged to seek technically competent help—usually from a physician. It is important to remember that these are *society's* expectations; the patient may or may not live up to them.

The obligation to want and to try to get well has been associated with the expectation that the sick role usually will be transient. Since society at large and the patient's family in particular can be expected to demand that the patient want and try to get better, it is tempting to conclude that the patient who, because of secondary gain or strong regressive dependency needs, "refuses" to get well is in conflict with society or his family. Where this conflict does exist the patient's behavior can be understood as resistance to the social norms, defiance, and aggressive control of the persons in his immediate environment. The emphasis here is on the patient's position as a deviant member of society, and the psychiatrist tends to focus on the patient and ask, "What is wrong with *him*"?

In more than a few cases, however, what appears as deviant or defiant behavior may really be compliant. There are a significant number of instances where family members neither expect the patient to get well nor do they genuinely desire improvement. In these situations we should not speak of the obligation to want to get well but rather of the obligation to remain sick.

The hospital, as a social institution, provides more than a

convenient and technically well-equipped place for treating the sick; it is a place where patients are expected to adopt the sick role. Here again, most often the patient is put under the obligation to want and to try to get well. However, just as with some families, there are also situations where the medical or nursing staff obliges the patient to remain sick. Further, as Weiner has reported, at times fellow patients may be the source of pressure on a particular patient to remain sick.

If the patient, his family, and the hospital staff are united in their contentment with the patient's sick role, the psychiatric consultant may not be called in. The patient will be labeled "chronic" and no psychosocial problem will be seen. However, when the patient's maintenance of the sick role conflicts with the expectations of the medical or nursing staff, the patient may be labeled a "management problem" and the aid of a psychiatrist may be enlisted. It is here that the consultant may find it helpful to assess the position of the family. What is sometimes found is that the patient and his family are in a stable equilibrium around his sick role; both the patient and the family gratify their needs through the "sickness."

There are undoubtedly a variety of circumstances which can bring about this stable equilibrium which the family promotes by obliging the patient to remain sick. Some of these circumstances are obvious—for example, when an illness brings a pension or compensation or when illness removes a patient from a very acute and obvious family crisis. We shall discuss some of the less apparent and more subtle changes in family relationships which may be reflected by the family demands that the patient remain ill.

REPORT OF CASES

Case 1. This patient, a 46-year-old white male, was admitted to the hospital after suffering a cerebral vascular accident which left him with a complete right hemiplegia and severe motor aphasia. Speech therapy progressed to the point where he could with some difficulty utter long sentences; through the efforts of physical therapy he was able to walk with the aid of a brace and cane and to climb stairs with considerable confidence.

He began to spend weekends at home and, with assistance from his wife, he was able to manage the visits quite adequately. About the time that the staff began to discuss discharge plans with the patient and his wife, ominous signs appeared. Following a long weekend at home, the patient's wife reported that he had been "worse than he was in several months." He had seemed annoyed at everyone and had complained more than was usual. During the next few months his behavior deteriorated to the point where he refused to eat, did not participate in physical therapy, and ultimately became mute and apparently unresponsive to his surroundings. He was confined to bed or a cardiac chair. However, at least early in this period, the mutism was interrupted by outbursts of psychotic speech, and at unpredictable times he would smile or grunt at certain personnel. Occasionally, he would spit his food at a nurse or kick a fellow patient. It was the general feeling of the staff that the patient was becoming increasingly depressed, possibly because of the realization that he was permanently disabled. The patient and his case were presented to one of us (B. B.) at a weekly psychiatric conference. It was the psychiatrist's opinion that while depression may have been present, the predominant psychiatric problem was one of hostile negativism which had reached psychotic proportions.

Here, then, we have a patient who apparently was making a good recovery from his cerebral vascular accident and then became "uncooperative" to the point of hostile negative withdrawal.

The patient's wife was seen for several interviews by the social worker (R. D'E.), following which the psychiatrist (B. B.) saw the patient, the wife, and the daughter in family therapy sessions until the wife broke off the contact. With these interviews, we were able to investigate the family's contribution to the patient's illness behavior.

The A family consisted of the patient, his wife, a son who was away at college, and a daughter who attended high school. The patient had supported the family as an independent salesman but his business had become increasingly poor in the year prior to his illness. The wife had always put a high value on material goods and she felt inferior to other members of her family who had a higher standard of living than she. Further, she felt that her husband had no respect for her needs or desires. The daughter was in constant war with her mother while the patient had remained aloof from their quarrels. The mother always spoke of the son as having no problems and she seemed quite content to have him safely away at the university.

During the early part of Mr. A's illness, the family seemed genuinely interested in his progress and the wife participated actively in helping the patient perform his exercise. During this time, also, the wife found it necessary to take over the business and it began to prosper. With her emerging sense of independence and self-sufficiency, her attitude toward the patient's illness changed. The interaction between the patient and his wife was put quite dramatically and succinctly by the daughter in one of our family meetings. We had been discussing whether the patient could sit in a wheelchair. The wife insisted that this would be impossible—the patient was "too sick." Referring then to his mutism and stubbornness, the daughter said

In a way I think I know how he would feel . . . I mean sitting there getting mad . . . I think he feels now a lot of resentment because we're talking about him and he can't tell us what he's feeling, he can't tell us if we're exaggerating or he can't defend himself . . . because maybe he's resentful, because she (the wife) took over his business and she's doing well and that he can't be out there doing it and she's supporting the family now. She's more or less wearing the pants in the family and he's just, you know, sitting here, and maybe he resents that a lot too and in that way . . . maybe in a way it helped not to make his progress fast. Maybe he was trying to keep himself back a little, by not caring and not doing anything. And maybe he doesn't want to tell my mother, and he feels that she seems to be doing all right by herself. This is why he was holding back and he wasn't showing any progress and maybe he was doing it purposely, and I felt that my mother was part of the reason why because she was, well, she was doing everything . . . and doing *his* job, and in a way I felt resentment for her because I thought she was part of the cause of it.

The daughter's statements, while expressive of her own role in the many family conflicts, had much truth in them.

Indeed, on the patient's last few home visits before his clinical course changed for the worse, the wife had shown him how independent she was and had even made a point of deciding to take him out on the road with her, but then, "realizing that this would be too tiring for him," she left him home.

The wife treated the patient as if she expected him to remain ill. She fought quite bitterly against the suggestion that the patient come to the family meetings in a wheelchair rather than in a cardiac chair, and she expressed surprise and objections to every suggestion that the patient not be treated as a complete invalid. She would lean over and chuck the patient under the chin calling him "Babe." She said

I mean isn't it logical that when a man gets sick like this, this is the natural thing especially when he's helpless . . . when a man becomes helpless and a mother (sic) . . . and a woman has to treat him like . . . like a child . . . do the same things that she would for a child, don't you automatically fall into the mother pattern? It's as if you had a baby . . . and it's having another child again you do the same things that you would for a child. So for your own pleasure (sic) is . . . he's not my flesh and blood and yet he is . . . you get that same feeling—you automatically, I think, lose the husband and wife feeling and you take on this other type of feeling.

The patient's response to this was a pervasive and apparently resentful helplessness and lack of apparent reaction which was most pronounced with respect to his wife.

When the patient had first become ill, his wife had genuinely attempted to help him recover; however, when she saw that his recovery would be limited and that she was destined to have even less of a provider as a husband, she apparently mobilized her own assertive and independent capacities and found to her delight that she could successfully take over his functions. At this time, she became reluctant to relinquish her new found gains (both materially and psychologically) and her chief interest seemed to be to carve out some sort of independent life for herself. Her husband was safely "put away" in a hospital because he was "sick"; her son was away at college, and she was attempting to marry off her daughter. In addition, by obliging him to remain sick (under the guise of maternal concern and solicitude), she was destroying him in the same sense that some parents foster the destruction of their sociopathic children by their "concern." The patient's incapacity probably gratified his wife's angry competitive impulses and her resentment at the "hard life" she had had before her husband's illness.

The patient probably saw his illness and his family situation as a threat to his own sense of masculinity. This must have played a part in provoking his regression to the stubborn, silent, defiant state. However, it becomes quite clear that the patient's negativism was not only defiant; in a very real sense he was complying with his wife's wishes. He was abdicating his right to assume the masculine role in the family and acceding to her wish to have him remain sick and infantilized. Thus, what appears on the one hand to have been a hostile struggle between husband and wife can also be viewed as a state of equilibrium.

The obligation that a family may place upon one of its members to remain ill does not always arise during an acute illness; in many cases the fact that one person is ill may have brought the spouses together in the first place. There are many women, for example, who marry chronically ill men with the aim of nursing them, but not nursing them back to health. This situation is described in the following case.

Case 2.   Mr. B was a man with a life-long passive and feminine orientation. His feminine tendencies were graphically illustrated by his tattooes; over the right nipple was tattooed a chubby girl's smiling face labeled "sweet" while over the left nipple a pouting girl bore the label of "sour."

The patient's renal disease was known to both him and his wife at the time of their marriage, and this knowledge fit in well with their conception of their respective roles. The wife was a steady and reliable worker who performed the instrumental tasks, she provided the family income. By contrast, the patient cooked the meals for the family. The wife expressed her satisfaction with this state of affairs by saying "people around here are funny, they can't understand how my husband's home and I work—because none of these people work—they just sit and talk and have coffee all day. I couldn't do that . . . I love to work—I get tired, I admit, but I would never quit." Although the patient had made several half-hearted attempts at working, his wife discouraged him by pointing out that any kind of work would get him too tired. Except for cooking, there seemed to be little else for the patient to do in his family but to "be the sick one." The wife was also the integrative-supportive member of the household; she did most of the housework and it was she to whom the two daughters, age 16 and 14 came for help and advice. The husband described his daily activities largely around feeling tired and being sick.

Within the family framework, the patient's sickness also served as a vehicle for expression of his anger. Whenever he was out with his wife socially, he would get "short of breath" or have an urge to move his bowels. These symptoms disappeared when they returned home. The wife was annoyed at the severe limitations this put on her social activities. However, she "understood" that these limitations were "unavoidable" because of the patient's sickness. At specific times when the family situation caused the patient to get even more acutely angry, this anger was quickly converted into symptoms of "sickness" which at times "required" hospitalization. For example, the daughter's boyfriend served as a point of friction between the patient and his wife. Although the patient disliked the boyfriend, the wife invited him to have dinner with them. As the patient reported, "I didn't care for the idea but to save an argument, I let him go in the house— we had dinner together and—like I say I don't know whether that brought that particular thing (an attack of nausea and vomiting) on or not, but it seemed so. I mean . . . I don't know, but like I say the following day *I was ready to go to the hospital and I did go to the hospital.*" With this hospitalization there was no chemical evidence of fluctuations in the state of the patient's renal disease, and the symptoms disappeared immediately upon hospitalization. The probable diagnosis was a conversion reaction and in retrospect, the internists felt that the hospitalization had not been indicated. The hospitalization inconvenienced the wife but once again, she saw this not so much as an expression of the patient's anger but as a necessary part of her life being married to a "sick man." Thus, the patient and his wife were prone to seize upon the sick role not only as a means of preserving their preferred roles in life but also as a means of avoiding potential angry conflict in the family.

In other cases, not only the family but also the physician and other staff members may oblige the patient to remain ill. This can particularly be seen on chronic wards where some patients are "good" patients and become fixtures on the ward. Sometimes the physicians and nurses may start out with a vigorous therapeutic regimen but may become discouraged with the patient's lack of responsiveness. This attitude on the part of the staff can convey to the patient the expectation that he is to remain chronically ill. The patient may receive the message that he is obliged to remain sick from the whole staff or from one part of the staff (such as a physician or some members of the nursing staff). This situation is illustrated in the following case.

Case 3. A 51-year-old man had had multiple infarcts resulting in the amputation of both of his legs and a cerebral vascular accident with some weakness of his arms and hands and a mild aphasia. He had been married late in life and had a wife and 7-year-old son at home. He was presented to the consultant since it was his physician's opinion that he should not go home on visits. The physician said, "I suspect that he will remain here as a patient. I should appreciate your talking with the wife since she needs some support with this decision since she feels quite guilty about not taking him home." The physician was particularly concerned because, although the patient had progressed to the point when he could have managed home visits, the doctor felt that the young son would be disturbed by the presence of his crippled father at home. Further, the physician was impressed with the unpredictability of the patient's illness and with his own inability to take any decisive steps to forestall further infarcts. The patient was described as "weepy and mildly depressed." His progress in speech therapy and physical therapy had leveled off at about the time that the physician had made it known that the patient would not be allowed home on weekend visits. Prior to that time, however, he had shown adequate progress.

The wife, indeed, was a guilty person; she felt guilty not only because the husband was not coming home but also because the husband was ill altogether. She was quite incapable of making her own decisions and depended upon others such as the physician to outline a course of action for her.

The physician was encouraged to explore some of the factors which led him to keep the patient in the sick role to a degree greater than that necessitated by his illness. He was quickly able to realize the lack of medical logic behind his prohibition and he began allowing the patient to go home for passes. Shortly thereafter, the patient appeared less depressed, the wife was less overtly guilty, and the patient once again made strides toward his rehabilitation.

COMMENT

It is interesting to examine how situations in which there is an obligation upon the patient to remain sick can eventuate in a request for psychiatric help. In our experiences, the request for psychiatric help often results from a conflict of obligations which are put on the patient. In the first case, Mr. A was complying with his wife's request to remain sick, but at the same time was confronted by the physician and hospital staff with a very serious request to get well. What was compliance with the wife was defiance of the staff. The staff felt that a conflict existed, but it was unable to accurately identify it; psychiatric aid was sought. By way of contrast, in the case of Mr. C it was the physician who had placed upon the patient the obligation to remain in the sick role whereas the wife and the patient could not comfortably accept this role. Once again the conflict of obligations occurred. It is interesting that a major reason for referral of this case was "to support the wife" in a decision to commit the patient to the sick and hospitalized role.

In the ordinary course of events, patient B might never have come to the attention of the psychiatrist. At home there were no striking conflicts of obligation. His hospitalizations (at times of temporary family crises) were usually self-limited, and as the anger abated the patient "spontaneously recovered" and the wife was quite willing to have him home again. The physicians, knowing that the illness would be fatal, did not oblige the patient to attempt to relinquish the sick role. In this case, Mr. B came to our attention as a part of a random sample for another research project. This situation can occasionally pose a serious problem on "chronic" medical wards. Without the conflict of obligations, no problems may be seen and chronicity may be perpetuated. Where psychiatrists make periodic rounds on medical and surgical wards they may be able to detect these situations; when the consultant must be "invited in," the problem may be overlooked.

In the light of our cases which illustrate that people in the patient's immediate milieu may oblige the patient to remain ill, we may ask whether these situations directly contradict Parsons' criteria for the sick role. Parsons has emphasized that the sick role is considered legitimate "so long as it is clearly recognized that it is intrinsically an undesirable state, to be recovered from as expeditiously as possible." We have seen that our patients are told that their sickness is legitimate and that they *must not* recover from their state as soon as possible. This "difference" from Parsons' theory is more apparent than real and depends upon the level of analysis. When one talks to the patient, one hears that he would prefer to recover as soon as possible. Likewise, on superficial conversation with members of the family (and the hospital staff) one also learns that the sickness is felt to be undesirable and "we are doing everything possible to help the patient recover." Most often on a conscious level this is true; the family believes that it is a victim of circumstances and the staff talks about a "chronic" patient. On this level, they join forces with the institutional mores of society which Parsons was describing. However, as psychiatrists, we realize that people may have motives of which they are not so fully aware and that these motives may conflict with the conscious desires. Obliging a husband to remain sick goes so against the social institutions that it is not surprising that a wife would hide this desire from both herself and others and replace it with a felt desire to have the patient recover. What emerges is a compromise formation. Thus, a wife may express concern, sympathy, overprotectiveness as if she wanted him to improve, but at the same time she may clearly convey to him the underlying feeling that sickness is what is expected. She says to him, "I would like you to get well and I will do everything possible, but I expect that you will remain sick (that is, I want you to remain sick)." Likewise, as in case C the staff may say, "we are doing everything to help you overcome your disability, but medical judgment dictates that you should remain an invalid." We have already noted in case A how these conflicting messages are similar to those given to sociopathic children by their parents. In another sense, they are similar to the double-blind as described by Bateson et al. The patient likewise reacts with a double reaction. He says, "I know you want me to get well and I too want to get well; isn't it unfortunate that I can't (that is, don't worry, I won't get well)." Whereas the wife (as in case A) may be expressing simultaneous love and destructive wishes, the patient simultaneously can express his hostile defiance and his compliance.

If it can be seen that a particular "uncooperative patient" not only is reacting in terms of his own passivity or defiance but also in response to a clear obligatory message given to him by members of his family, it would seem logical that the therapeutic approach be directed not only at the patient but at the whole family. To date, our experience with the therapy of families showing this type of equilibrium has been more enlightening to us than encouraging. This is understandable when we realize that a state of equilibrium on the basis of the patient's illness has been reached between the patient and the person obliging him to remain ill, and that in order to produce change one first has to destroy this equilibrium. There is great resistance to this on the part of both partners. Thus, in our preliminary attempts at family therapy, we have encountered a high degree of spontaneous termination. We have been somewhat more successful when the equilibrium has been more recently arrived at or when the psychosocial crisis in the family was relatively self-limited. With a nidus of actual physical illness for the family to focus on, it is often difficult to get the participants to consider the family's equilibrium as an illness. This problem has been reported also by Jackson and Weakland in their treatment of the families of schizophrenic patients. The family is supported in its use of the patient's sick role as a means of maintaining equilibrium by our social institutions which make this role legitimate. Further, the fact that family therapy is not a usual (institutionalized) form of treatment for patients hospitalized on medical or surgical wards probably constitutes another barrier to success. Much work remains to be done in order to provide us with techniques to break up this equilibrium.

SUMMARY

It is generally assumed that persons in the immediate milieu of the patient on the medical or surgical wards oblige the patient to want and to try to get better. There are circumstances, however, where the family and/or the hospital staff conveys a double message to the patient. While superficially telling the patient to improve, they may clearly indicate their expectation that he remain sick. When the psychiatric consultant is asked to help in the management of an "uncooperative" patient, he must be aware that this noncooperation may not be only defiance; on another level it may be compliance with the demands of others. The features of this situation leading to the request for psychiatric assistance are discussed, as are the problems encountered when family therapy is used to attempt to break up these situations.

Institutionalism in Mental Hospitals

J. K. WING

INTRODUCTION

The term "institutionalism" can presumably be used to describe any behaviour which is evoked in an individual by the social pressures of an institution. In a wider context, Merton (1957) has described five types of individual adaptation to cultural values—conformity, innovation, ritualism, retreatism, and rebellion—which could be used as a basis for systematic investigation. No doubt other syndromes could also be delineated. Social organizations such as the Government, the Church or the Family are as legitimately called institutions as are orphanages or convents. Many writers, however, have referred particularly to a form of behavioural reaction which is said to occur frequently among individuals who have remained for prolonged periods in certain types of segregated community. Bettelheim & Sylvester (1948), for example, described an institution in which a rigid, comprehensive and impersonal regime allowed no scope for individual decisions on the part of the inmate children and, demanding only their compliance, led to emotional apathy, lack of spontaneity, and an incapacity for active adjustment to events which were commonplace to non-institutionalized children. Similar terms have been used to describe the effects of prisons, tuberculosis sanatoria, mental hospitals, and homes for old people, and Titmuss (1958) has indicated the same tendencies in some general hospitals. The effects of

FROM the *British Journal of Social and Clinical Psychology* 1 (1962) 38–51. Reprinted by permission of the author and the publisher.

prolonged incarceration in segregated communities have been described in detail in numerous novels and descriptive works, again with remarkable agreement on such details of the syndrome as apathy, resignation, dependence, depersonalization, and reliance on fantasy. It is this limited concept of "institutionalism" which provided the starting-point for the present work.

No doubt because of the difficult methodological problems involved, few of the studies so far published have described the systematic collection of empirical data which could serve as a basis for firm conclusions as to the nature and origin of institutionalism. Before reporting a preliminary attempt to provide such data, some of the factors involved in investigating institutionalism will be considered in detail. In particular, three variables have obvious relevance: (a) The actual social pressures to which an individual is exposed after admission to an institution, whether general—common to all institutions—or specific to one particular kind. (b) The pattern of susceptibility or resistance to various types of institutional pressure which the individual possesses when he is first admitted. (c) The length of time that the inmate is exposed to the pressures.

Each of these variables will be discussed, firstly, in the general context of all institutions, irrespective of type, and secondly, in the specific context of the mental hospital.

(a) The Social Pressures of an Institution

Erving Goffman (1958) calls certain segregated communities "total institutions," and lists a number of features which they have in common. The staff and inmates have fundamentally different points of view, and may come to perceive each other in narrow, hostile stereotypes. There is great social distance between the two sides and little movement between them. Decisions about admission and discharge are made by authority and the individual has little say in them. The amount of contact with non-institutional life is strictly rationed and is looked upon as a privilege. The inmates sleep, play and work in one place, and an overall rational plan guides all behaviour. Even the smallest detail, such as when an inmate shall bath or cut his nails, may be decided for him. Social experience is reduced to a uniform dullness. The inmate is no longer looked upon as a father, or an employee, or a customer, or as a member of numerous specialized social groups, and his ability to play everyday social roles may atrophy from disuse. He does not practise travelling on buses, or spending money, or choosing food or clothes. His relationships with the outside world are reduced to a minimum.

These are features of "bad" institutions—authoritarian, custodial, and deadening—and they are the reason for the recent reaction against the use of the institution for solving or alleviating social problems, as Titmuss (1959) has pointed out. "No such swing of opinion away from the *good* institution can be discerned: the effective general hospital for the acutely ill, the public school and other socially approved forms of institutional care. But these have been experienced and remembered only by a minority; for most people institutional life has spelt little besides ugliness, cheapness, and restricted liberties."

Many of the general factors which total institutions are said to have in common may certainly be seen in mental hospitals, and all the features of behaviour and attitudes which make up the syndrome of institutionalism may readily be found among long-stay mental patients (Belknap, 1956; Caudill, 1958; Goffman, 1959). However, in addition to these general pressures, institutions often have an educating, treating, or reforming function which takes a wide variety of specific forms according to the ostensible purpose of the institution. Such methods include the re-education of a persistent offender (Scott, 1960), the extraction of confessions, or the conversion of prisoners-of-war to a different political point of view (Schein, 1956). The effects of such positive pressures have to be disentangled from the effects of the more general routines mentioned earlier since they may advance or retard the development of institutionalism.

The specific features of treatment in mental hospitals are difficult to allow for individually. They include electrically-induced convulsions, prefrontal leucotomy and other brain operations, insulin comas, and treatment with various types of drugs. Social treatments include group psychotherapy, re-education through contact with a "therapeutic milieu," and planned occupational therapy, though these have often not been extensively used until very recently, and long-term patients will not have had the benefit of such methods during most of their stay in hospital. Dietary deficiencies and the physiological results of underactivity may also have affected the clinical picture in past years (Kety, 1959).

It is probably safe to say that most patients who have been continuously resident for more than two years in a mental hospital will have been exposed to many of the general features of "total" institutions, and that the presence of features specific to mental hospitals is unlikely to have retarded much the process of institutionalism.

(b) Susceptibility to Institutional Pressures

Persons sent to prison, mentally ill patients, individuals suffering from tuberculosis, orphans, prisoners-of-war and refugees are all in their different ways unrepresentative of the general population of a country, and they take with them, if they are admitted to an institution, their own specific characteristics. However, some are more likely to be admitted than others and there may be general factors which make admission to any institution more probable. Those who have not built up strong ties in an outside community through marriage or work or family or other interests; those who are vulnerable because of poverty or age or social position; those who have never been concerned with problems of personal liberty and decision-taking; those in whom social relationships induce anxiety or discomfort and who prefer a social environment where interaction can be minimal—all these may have an increased liability to admission, and their chance of discharge later on may be reduced. Thus there may be, for various reasons, a state of susceptibility to institutionalism which is present when the individual first enters the segregated community, so that, at its most extreme, a person may show dependence on the institution, and apathy about leaving, very shortly after admission (Ellenberger, 1960). The essence of the concept of institutionalism, as so far discussed, is that exposure to the social pressures of the institution has brought about a change in the individual's behaviour and attitudes: but the limiting case occurs where such behaviour is already present in embryo before admission. If a great many such people are admitted, the apparently high prevalence of "institutionalism," compared with that in another community, may be misleading.

So far as mental hospitals are concerned there is another problem. All the inmates are there because they are 'ill' in some way. Since over half the patients in mental hospitals (and over three-quarters of those who have been in hospital more than two years) are suffering from schizophrenia, it will be convenient to limit discussion to this disease. The question arises how far the typical symptoms of the illness (in which shallowness of emotional response and lack of motivation are common symptoms even when the patient has never been admitted to hospital) can be distinguished from the aspects of behaviour and attitudes which are said to be characteristic of institutionalism. Schizophrenic patients, by reason of their numbers and prolonged residence, acquire, transmit, and partially determine the peculiar culture of the hospital community (Sommer, 1959). The problem of institutionalism in mental hospitals has become therefore, in large measure, the problem of the long-term management of schizophrenia.

Thus it is important to try to discover whether any deteriorating effect of institutional procedures can be demonstrated in schizophrenic patients. Such deterioration might take place either in aspects of behaviour and in attitudes which would be regarded by physicians as part of the illness, irrespective of social setting (for example, marked blunting of affect, disordered speech, delusions or hallucinations), or in aspects of behaviour and in attitudes which could reasonably be regarded as part of a syndrome of institutionalism even in people who were not ill (for example, dependence on the institution, apathy about leaving, lack of interest in events outside, lack of competence in extramural activities, resignation towards the institutional mode of life, and so on). Since, logically, either of these two sets of factors may vary independently of the other, any investigation into the effects of prolonged institutional pressures should differentiate between them as clearly as possible, though some overlapping cannot be avoided. (In particular, apathy and flatness of affect, unrealistic ideas about the future and delusions, must overlap.)

The classical view, that the familiar "end-state" seen in long-hospitalized schizophrenics is an inevitable consequence of the deterioration inherent in the disease, has probably never been held, in pure form, by any psychiatrist. Nevertheless, it has in part determined a good deal of clinical thinking on the subject. The opposite, equally extreme view, that the end-state is solely dependent on the social environment, has probably never been held by any sociologist, though some have seemed to approach such a position. A moderate medical viewpoint has been stated by Lewis (1953). "The concept of disease has physiological and psychological components but no essential social ones. In examining it we cannot ignore social considerations, because they may be needed for the assessment of physiological and psychological adequacy, but we are not bound to consider whether behaviour is socially deviant: though illness may lead to such behaviour, there are many forms of social deviation which are not illness, many forms of illness which are not social deviation." Wootton (1959) has recently reinforced this view. The important point is that, although the social environment may influence the onset and course of the disease, illness and environment remain logically distinct: each may vary independently of the other.

(c) Length of Exposure to Institutional Pressures

A short-term deprivation of liberty, even with complete and perhaps humiliating change of routine, is unlikely to have much lasting effect on the average individual (for example, during a brief stay in a general hospital) unless there is some kind of susceptibility. On the other hand, many years in a "maximum-security" prison, exposed to a rigidly monotonous regime which allowed no opportunity for individual responsibility in deciding everyday behaviour, would surely affect most people in some way, though a number of resistant individuals would no doubt be found. One would expect, therefore, that the longer a person had been exposed to such routines the more likely he would be to show traits of institutionalism. On the other hand, specific environmental pressures of various kinds might accelerate or slow down the process of change, and determine its direction. Since a long-term study of changes in behaviour and attitudes over many years has obvious practical disadvantages, it might appear sensible to compare individuals who had been resident in a total institution for varying periods of time. There is a serious objection to this method, however, unless the effect of selection can be allowed for. Not only may individuals succumb immediately to institutional pressures (with an exacerbation of symptoms or the appearance of institutionalized behaviour patterns) but there may be a selective effect of certain social characteristics, such as marital and occupational status, on length of stay. This is certainly true of schizophrenic patients in mental hospitals (Norris, 1956; Brooke, 1957). Brown (1960*a*) has shown that schizophrenics who were visited during the first two months after admission in 1950 had a significantly greater chance of leaving hospital than those who were not. No doubt a similar selective effect could be found in those who were apathetic on admission, which could partly account for any higher proportion of apathetic patients in the longer-stay groups.

Fortunately, this factor can be allowed for to some extent, since the chance of discharge after two years' continuous stay in hospital was not, until recently, a very considerable one, and a large increase in, for example, the proportion of apathetic patients in the longer-stay groups could not be explained in such a way (Kramer, 1955; Brown, 1960*b*). In order to allow to some extent for the effect of increasing age, it would be desirable also to omit from the study patients who had reached the age of sixty.

In summary, so far as general features go, most mental hospitals are likely to exhibit many of the features of "total" institutions, and their specific features are not likely to obscure the study of institutionalism, particularly if recently admitted patients, who may have been exposed to less restrictive regimes, are excluded. In order to avoid the complexities introduced by studying many different diagnostic categories, interest should be focused particularly on schizophrenic patients, who form three-quarters of the long-stay group. Aspects of behaviour which are characteristic of the illness irrespective of its social setting should be studied separately from aspects of behaviour which are thought to be typical of "total" institutions whether the inmates are mentally ill or not. Since schizophrenic patients with certain social characteristics are likely to be discharged within two years of admission, and since the chance of discharge for the remainder does not rise markedly thereafter, deterioration, if present, should be demonstrated in the latter group. A suitable method would be to compare groups of patients who had been resident for varying periods of time.

This kind of investigation would not take into account the possibility of relatively rapid changes for the better or for the worse, either in schizophrenic symptoms or in institutional behaviour and attitudes. These would be more suitably investigated in specific experiments. Only a limited hypothesis could be tested—that there is a gradual deterioration, over many years, in the attitudes and behaviour of schizophrenic patients who are aged fifty-nine and under and who have already spent at least two years in the mental hospital. The present investigation is not concerned with other mental illnesses, nor with other types of behavioural reaction (e.g. neurotic or antisocial) in the inmates of institutions.

PRESENT INVESTIGATION

Standard data were collected about random samples of half the male chronic schizophrenic populations of two London mental hospitals. Only male patients, under 60 years of age, were selected. Lists of names were drawn up in alphabetical order, by wards, of those said unequivocally in the case records to be schizophrenic. Every second patient on these lists was interviewed and a schedule of information was completed by the ward charge nurse. The information collected, apart from age and length of present stay, was of three kinds:

(a) Ratings of symptoms made after a psychiatric examination by the investigator. The symptoms rated were emotional blunting, poverty of speech, incoherence of speech, delusions and hallucinations. Each was rated on a 5-point scale (1, no disorder; 2, minimal; 3, moderate; 4, severe; 5, very severe). On the basis of this material, the patients were divided into three groups:

  (i) Moderately ill (a rating of 3 or less in each category).
 (ii) Severely ill with "florid" symptoms (a rating of 4 or 5 on incoherence of speech or delusions, irrespective of other ratings).
(iii) Severely ill without "florid" symptoms (all remaining patients).

In this way three clinically well-recognizable groups were obtained. The reliability of the clinical ratings, and of the classification derived from them, was investigated in detail (Wing, 1961) and was found to be satisfactory.

(b) At the same interview, a number of standard questions were asked about how strongly the patient wanted to leave hospital and what his plans for the future were. Ratings of attitude to discharge were made on a 5-point scale (1, keenly wishes to leave; 2, leaves decision to discretion of doctor, relative, etc.; 3, very vague or ambivalent about leaving; 4, seemingly indifferent; 5, definitely prefers to stay in hospital). The correlation coefficient for two psychiatrists independently rating the same random sample of 25 men and 25 women, all schizophrenic and long-hospitalized, was 0.83. Plans for the future were also rated on a 5-point scale (1, definite, realistic plans; 2, fairly definite plans, on balance realistic; 3, fairly definite plans, on balance unrealistic; 4, fairly definite plans, quite unrealistic; 5, no plans at all).

(c) The senior charge nurse of each ward was asked to observe each patient's behaviour over seven days and then complete a rating schedule about him (Wing, 1960a). From this schedule two scores were derived. The first represented social withdrawal and was composed of items concerning conversation, degree of interaction, interests, care of appearance, slowness and underactivity (range of scores $+ 8$ to $- 24$). The second represented socially embarrassing behaviour and was composed of items concerning overactivity, irritability, bizarre mannerisms, talking and laughing to self and abnormal speech content (range of scores 0 to $- 32$). These scores were completely independent of the interview data. Reliability, determined in preliminary work, was satisfactory for the social withdrawal score: during extensive testing, r varied from 0.73 to 0.87. Reliability, on the other score, was satisfactory as between nurses ($r = 0.67$–0.77) but more variable between different occasions of rating ($r = 0.38$–0.91).

RESULTS

For the purposes of comparison, the data from the two hospitals (in which the main variables were similarly distributed) were combined.

1. Attitudes to Discharge and Plans for the Future

The distribution of attitude ratings in five length-of-stay groups is shown in Tables 1 and 2. When the group of patients who have been in hospital less than two years is omitted (because of the considerations mentioned earlier), it is clear that there is still a marked concentration of the less satisfactory attitudes in the longer-stay groups. Twenty-nine per cent of patients who have been in hospital from two to five years have a fairly definite desire to leave, and 34 per cent wish to stay. The equivalent proportions of patients who have been in hospital over twenty years are 3 per cent and 83 per cent.

The position with respect to plans for the future is similar. The relationship is not dependent upon age. Table 3 shows the numbers and proportions of patients, within three age-groups, who have some desire to leave hospital (a rating of 1, 2 or 3). There is a significant association with length of stay in each case.

Length of illness (from time of first admission to hospital for mental illness), as opposed to length of stay, is more difficult to allow for because the two variables are highly correlated. However, within the group of patients who have been ill from ten to twenty years, there is still a highly significant association between length of stay and attitude to discharge (see Table 4).

2. Clinical Classification of Schizophrenic Symptoms

Table 5 shows that there is no overall relationship between the clinical classification of the patients and their length of stay ($\chi^2 = 1.52$, d.f. $= 6$, $p = > 0.05$). Members of the three clinical subgroups tend to have different attitudes to dis-

TABLE 1. Attitude to Discharge by Length of Stay in Hospital

	\<1:11		2–4:11		5–9:11		10–19:11		20 +		Total over 2 years	
Rating of attitude to discharge	N	%	N	%	N	%	N	%	N	%	N	%
1 and 2 (Definite wish to leave)	36	50.7	12	29.3	13	23.6	6	11.3	1	2.8	32	17.3
3 (Vague wish to leave)	17	23.9	15	36.6	14	25.5	6	11.3	5	13.9	40	21.6
4 and 5 (Indifferent or wish to stay)	18	25.4	14	34.2	28	50.9	41	77.4	30	83.3	113	61.1
Total	71	100.0	41	100.1	55	100.0	53	100.0	36	100.0	185	100.0

TABLE 2. Plans for the Future by Length of Stay in Hospital

	\<1:11		2–4:11		5–9:11		10–19:11		20 +		Total over 2 years	
Rating of plans for the future	N	%	N	%	N	%	N	%	N	%	N	%
1 and 2 (Realistic plans)	33	46.5	17	41.5	12	21.8	6	11.3	3	8.3	38	20.5
3 and 4 (Unrealistic plans)	14	19.7	9	22.0	11	20.0	10	18.9	4	11.2	34	18.4
5 (No rateable plans)	24	33.8	15	36.6	32	58.2	37	69.8	29	80.6	113	61.1
Total	71	100.0	41	100.1	55	100.0	53	100.0	36	100.1	185	100.0

TABLE 3. Attitudes to Discharge by Length of Stay, Within Three Age-groups

		Age				
		30–39		40–49		50–59
Length of stay	N	% with some wish to leave	N	% with some wish to leave	N	% with some wish to leave
$<$ 1:11	26	69.2	18	66.7	8 ⎫	
2–4:11	17	76.5	13	76.9	4 ⎬	54.6
5–9:11	24	37.5	17	58.8	10 ⎭	
10–19:11	23 ⎫	16.7	17 ⎫	14.8	13	38.5
20 +	1 ⎭		10 ⎭		25	20.0
χ^2		20.7		22.1		6.1
p		< 0.001		< 0.001		< 0.05

TABLE 4. Attitudes to Discharge by Length of Stay
(considering only patients *first* admitted to hospital between ten and twenty years previously)

Length of stay	N	Percentage with some wish to leave
$<$ 1:11	13	84.6
2–19:11	32	53.2
20 +	46	23.9

($\chi^2 = 17.3$, d.f. $= 2$, $p = < 0.001$)

charge, and the overall relationship is significant ($\chi^2 = 8.6$, d.f. $= 2$, $p = < 0.02$). However, although this tendency remains evident within each of the four length-of-stay groups, it is not statistically significant in any of them. On the other hand, the relationship between attitude and length of stay remains significant in each of the clinical subgroups.

3. Behaviour Ratings

The mean behavioural scores in four length-of-stay groups are shown in Table 6. Analysis of variance discloses no significant difference between the group means (e.g. for Social Withdrawal, $F = 0.93$, $p = > 0.05$).

TABLE 5. Attitude to Discharge by Clinical Grouping and Length of Stay

Clinical Groups	Length of stay									
	2–4:11		5–9:11		10–19:11		20 +		Total	
	N	% with some wish to leave	N	% with some wish to leave	N	% with some wish to leave	N	% with some wish to leave	N	% with some wish to leave
Moderately ill	13	84.6	14	50.0	18	33.3	10	30.0	55	49.1
Severely ill with "florid" symptoms	12	66.7	19	57.9	15	26.7	11	27.3	57	45.6
Severely ill without "florid" symptoms	16	50.0	22	40.9	20	10.0	15	0.0	73	26.0

TABLE 6. Social Behavior (Mean Scores) by Length of Stay in Hospital

Type of ward behaviour	Length of stay			
	2–4:11	5–9:11	10–19:11	20 +
Social withdrawal	− 4·1	− 5·5	− 3·5	− 6·0
Socially embarrassing behaviour	− 3·9	− 4·3	− 5·5	− 5·6

4. Confirmatory Study

In order to check the reliability of these results, and to increase the objectivity of the attitude rating, a further study was carried out in which all the male chronic schizophrenic patients of one of the hospitals were rated by the ward charge nurses on their behaviour during one week of observation. On this occasion the nurses were asked to tick on a check-list, for each patient, those items of behaviour which were noted during the week. They were also asked about the visitors the patients received, and the visits they made home.

The patients themselves were asked to select one of three items on a card, which described different attitudes towards leaving hospital. ((1) I want to leave as soon as possible, whatever the difficulties; (2) I want to leave sometime but there are a lot of problems; (3) I prefer to stay in hospital. Forty out of 132 patients were not able to say which of these alternatives they preferred. A few of those who made a choice seemed to do so at random, and some chose an item completely at variance with what they said, or with their current behaviour (nearly all the patients interviewed were under no form of legal restriction and could have left hospital at any time without formality). Nevertheless, the choices do show a significant association with length of stay, as is shown in Table 7. (Combining the second and third rows, $\chi^2 = 8.1$, d.f. = 2, $p = < 0.02$.)

TABLE 7. Self-rated Attitudes by Length of Stay in Hospital

Attitude to discharge	Length of stay							
	2–4:11		5–19:11		20 +		Total	
	N	%	N	%	N	%	N	%
Definitely wants to leave soon	13	72.2	24	47.1	7	30.4	44	47.8
Wants to leave one day	5	27.8	11	21.6	6	26.1	22	23.9
Prefers to stay	—	—	16	31.4	10	43.5	26	28.3
Total	18	100.0	51	100.1	23	100.0	92	100.0
Not able to say	7	—	27	—	6	—	40	—

The analysis of the behavioural check-list is presented in Table 8. Only one of the items shows any deviation from the expected frequency in the four length-of-stay groups. There is a significant increase in the proportion of patients laughing or talking out loud to themselves, with increase in length of stay ($\chi^2 = 13.4$, d.f. = 3, $p = < 0.01$).

There is a very highly significant relationship between length of stay and visiting, as shown in Table 9. The longer a patient has been in hospital, the less likely is he to receive visitors ($\chi^2 = 35.5$, d.f. = 4, $p = < 0.001$).

TABLE 8. Specific Items of Social Behaviour by Length of Stay in Hospital

Behavioural characteristic	Percentage of each length-of-stay group showing the characteristic				Total number showing characteristic
	2–4:11	5–9:11	10–19:11	20 +	
Mute and inaccessible	12.0	12.1	22.2	17.2	22
Passively withdrawn	44.0	42.4	37.8	58.6	59
Laughing or talking to self	32.0	39.4	57.8	75.9	69
Occasional restlessness or excitement	36.0	42.4	48.9	34.4	55
Violent, threatening or destructive	16.0	15.2	15.6	6.9	18
Liable to be incontinent, or needs washing or dressing	24.0	21.2	35.6	37.9	40
Extreme slowness or underactivity	32.0	24.2	24.4	27.6	35
Complete lack of interest (even in television)	32.0	24.2	37.8	34.5	43
Total number "at risk"	25	33	45	29	132

TABLE 9. Visiting by Length of Stay in Hospital

	Length of stay in hospital							
	2–9:11		10–19:11		20 +		Total	
	N	%	N	%	N	%	N	%
Goes home, or is visited regularly	43	74.1	16	35.6	3	10.3	62	47.0
Visited less than once a month. Does not go home	6	10.3	11	24.4	10	34.5	27	20.5
Never visited and never goes home	9	15.5	18	40.0	16	55.2	43	32.6
Total	58	99.9	45	100.0	29	100.0	132	100.0

DISCUSSION

It may be dangerous to infer a longitudinally-acting causal process from cross-sectional data. Nevertheless, that part of the hypothesis which predicts a gradual deterioration in attitudes with length of stay has not been disproved, as it might well have been. There is a progressive increase, with length of present stay, in the proportion of patients who appear apathetic about life outside hospital. This association is not wholly dependent on present age (in any case, patients over fifty-nine were not included in the study), nor on the length of time since the patient was first admitted for mental illness. Patients who had been in hospital for less than two years were omitted and the factor of selection (though still present to some extent) cannot account for the high relationship found. This relationship can be demonstrated in all three clinical groups—in fact it is most obvious in the large group of patients with severe blunting of emotional responsiveness and poverty of speech. The patients' self-ratings of attitude (though of somewhat doubtful validity) show a similar pattern. The hypothesis that there is a gradual change in attitude in patients who stay for prolonged periods in a mental hospital will therefore, for purposes of further discussion, be accepted.

The attitudes chosen for investigation are probably representative of a wider syndrome which may reasonably be termed 'institutionalism', many aspects of which were not measured. A hint as to one kind of factor which may be operating to produce this syndrome is given in Table 9, which shows the increasing lack of contact between patients and their relatives, with increase in length of stay. In a current research project, in which the effect of an Industrial Rehabilitation Unit (primarily for non-institutionalized disabled persons) on chronic schizophrenic men is being studied, their lack of competence in everyday activities which most people take for granted is very striking. The resulting aversion from everyday extramural life, and the attraction of the diminished responsibility which in-patient status allows, lies at the very heart of institutionalism.

No doubt the various factors described by Goffman as characteristic of total institutions operate to a greater or lesser extent in different establishments. In mental hospitals (even good ones, such as the two hospitals investigated here) the emphasis for the majority of inmates has been on a long stay, and a marked social isolation from the community. Schizophrenic patients may be more sensitive to such factors than inmates of other segregated communities, but this syndrome of institutionalism is presumably due mainly to similar pressures to those operating in other "total" institutions over long periods of time. It is therefore possible that something similar could be demonstrated in other long-stay establishments such as preventive-detention prisons or refugee camps, though no doubt different combinations of factors would produce differences in the syndromes of institutionalism found.

In marked contrast to these findings, very little relationship could be demonstrated between length of stay and symptoms of the illness, as manifested during a clinical examination, or in behaviour during a week of observation by a senior ward nurse. There is certainly no evidence of an inevitable clinical deterioration in the male schizophrenic population of the two mental hospitals studied, once they had been resident for two years. It is possible that more subtle measurements would have demonstrated a progressive increase in schizophrenic deficits with time, but from an overall clinical point of view, there were as many patients with marked flatness of affect and poverty of speech in the shorter- as in the longer-stay groups. Kleist (Fish, 1957) and Leonhard (1957; Fish, 1958) have shown, in detailed studies, that the leading symptom in 'true' chronic schizophrenic illnesses does not show much variation once the patient has been ill for ten years. A majority of the patients in the present study had been ill for many years before they had been admitted to hospital on the present occasion. "Deterioration," which is a firmly held clinical concept, may have taken place mainly during the first ten years of the illness, which remained relatively stable thereafter, as Kleist and Leonhard suggest. The present study can throw no light on whether such early deterioration occurred, nor to what extent it could have been prevented if a satisfactory social environment had been provided.

In addition to this limitation, it should also be emphasized that environmental stimuli may have effects which are relatively rapid in action. It has long been considered that catatonic motor symptoms (for example, rigidity of posture, apparently purposeless or impulsive movements, stereotyped mannerisms, etc.) are very markedly affected by the therapeutic regime adopted. The hospitals concerned in this survey, like all good modern mental hospitals, adopt a ward routine which minimises both the underactivity and the overactivity of such patients, and "typical" catatonics are now hardly to be seen. But if schizophrenics are placed in certain sorts of social environment, their symptoms may still be exacerbated, and the change may take place very quickly. Such effects, if they exist, would not, of course, be demonstrated by the present method of investigation.

Thus, "institutionalism," in the sense of a gradually acquired contentment in institutional life and apathy towards events outside hospital, does seem to be a factor of major importance even in good mental hospitals. "Deterioration," in the sense of a gradually increasing clinical deficit, cannot be demonstrated once the patient has been resident for two years. Relatively rapid 'fluctuations' in the clinical state, due to changes in the social environment, may occur, but would not be recorded using the present technique.

From the point of view of rehabilitation, a long-stay schizophrenic patient in these two mental hospitals may have two sorts of handicaps: the chronic symptoms which identify him as a schizophrenic and which limit his capacity for work and independent living ("primary disabilities"); and the handicaps which he has secondarily acquired during a prolonged stay in a semi-closed institution. In the latter case there is the problem of preventing the development of institutional attitudes, or of mitigating their effects. In the former case, there is the problem of providing a social setting in which, with skilled physiological and psychological treatments, schizophrenic symptoms will be minimised. Making such a distinction allows a more rational approach to social therapy, and a more realistic assessment of the benefits to be expected from it.

The recent development of multiple admissions of short duration, with adequate support during periods out of hospital, is bound to have a beneficial effect in preventing secondary handicaps, if it is carried out efficiently. The basic requirement is that residual primary dysfunctions which continue to handicap a schizophrenic after discharge from hospital should be recognized, and appropriate help given. In addition, social liability or socially embarrassing behaviour should not be allowed to reach a point at which the hospital's relationship with the community is likely to be damaged. The social isolation of mental hospital patients is due in part to the way in which they are perceived by the general public (Carstairs & Wing, 1958).

A healthy social environment in hospital will help to reduce both types of handicap to a minimum, though it will not necessarily cure schizophrenia. However, where attitudes have already become set in an institutional mould, as may be the case with 40 per cent or more of the chronic schizophrenic patients currently in mental hospital (even excluding those aged sixty and over), rehabilitation and resettlement present exceedingly difficult problems. In the days when few patients were expected to leave mental hospitals, the induction of such a state of mind had obvious advantages. Even now, the amenability of institutional schizophrenics is very striking compared with the relative intractability of acutely ill psychotics, and it can be used in rehabilitation, if not in resettlement. It is a grave handicap in those patients who are not ill enough to need further in-patient treatment, and it brings up all sorts of moral problems as to how far they should be pressed to change their attitudes. There is evidence that many handicapped schizophrenic patients can work reasonably well, and that some can maintain themselves, while living in hospital (Early, 1960). If their attitude has not finally crystallized into a determined wish to remain in hospital, they may eventually, with help, resettle and become self-supporting outside (Wing, 1960*b*).

Many suggestions have been put forward as to the kind of

social milieu which would favour the preservation of healthy attitudes and, at the same time, minimize schizophrenic symptoms. So far, the experimental work which alone can answer such problems is lacking.

I am indebted to Dr. A. B. Monro and Dr. R. K. Freudenberg, and to their staffs, for their co-operation and encouragement.

PART IV

Medical and Social Issues in the Field of Mental Illness

The social science point of view toward mental illness does not always merely supplement the medical point of view, but in some of its forms, contradicts it. This contradiction is represented most clearly in the work of the psychiatrist Thomas Szasz, whose "Myth of Mental Illness" is the first article in this section. In the next article, Szasz's argument that mental illness is a myth is criticized by Ausubel. In the short excerpt from Goffman's discussion of "normal deviants," a social structural framework is delineated. Lemert outlines a sociological theory of paranoia which integrates the perspectives of social structure and individual psychology. In the final selection, Erikson indicates some of the larger issues that connect deviance with the functioning of an on-going society.

The Myth of Mental Illness

THOMAS S. SZASZ

My aim in this essay is to raise the question "Is there such a thing as mental illness?" and to argue that there is not. Since the notion of mental illness is extremely widely used nowadays, inquiry into the ways in which this term is employed would seem to be especially indicated. Mental illness, of course, is not literally a "thing"—or physical object—and hence it can "exist" only in the same sort of way in which other theoretical concepts exist. Yet, familiar theories are in the habit of posing, sooner or later—at least to those who come to believe in them—as "objective truths" (or "facts"). During certain historical periods, explanatory conceptions such as deities, witches, and microorganisms appeared not only as theories but as self-evident *causes* of a vast number of events. I submit that today mental illness is widely regarded in a somewhat similar fashion, that is, as the cause of innumerable diverse happenings. As an antidote to the complacent use of the notion of mental illness—whether as a self-evident phenomenon, theory, or cause—let us ask this question: What is meant when it is asserted that someone is mentally ill?

In what follows I shall describe briefly the main uses to which the concept of mental illness has been put. I shall argue that this notion has outlived whatever usefulness it might have had and that it now functions merely as a convenient myth.

FROM *The American Psychologist* 15 (February 1960) 113–118. Reprinted by permission of the author and the publisher.

MENTAL ILLNESS AS A SIGN
OF BRAIN DISEASE

The notion of mental illness derives its main support from such phenomena as syphilis of the brain or delirious conditions—intoxications, for instance—in which persons are known to manifest various peculiarities or disorders of thinking and behavior. Correctly speaking, however, these are diseases of the brain, not of the mind. According to one school of thought, *all* so-called mental illness is of this type. The assumption is made that some neurological defect, perhaps a very subtle one, will ultimately be found for all the disorders of thinking and behavior. Many contemporary psychiatrists, physicians, and other scientists hold this view. This position implies that people *cannot* have troubles—expressed in what are *now called* "mental illnesses"—because of differences in personal needs, opinions, social aspirations, values, and so on. *All problems in living* are attributed to physicochemical processes which in due time will be discovered by medical research.

"Mental illnesses" are thus regarded as basically no different than all other diseases (that is, of the body). The only difference, in this view, between mental and bodily diseases is that the former, affecting the brain, manifest themselves by means of mental symptoms; whereas the latter, affecting other organ systems (for example, the skin, liver, etc.), manifest themselves by means of symptoms referable to those parts of the body. This view rests on and expresses what are, in my opinion, two fundamental errors.

In the first place, what central nervous system symptoms would correspond to a skin eruption or a fracture? It would *not* be some emotion or complex bit of behavior. Rather, it would be blindness or a paralysis of some part of the body. The crux of the matter is that a disease of the brain, analogous to a disease of the skin or bone, is a neurological defect, and not a problem in living. For example, a *defect* in a person's visual field may be satisfactorily explained by correlating it with certain definite lesions in the nervous system. On the other hand, a person's *belief*—whether this be a belief in

Christianity, in Communism, or in the idea that his internal organs are "rotting" and that his body is, in fact, already "dead"—cannot be explained by a defect or disease of the nervous system. Explanations of this sort of occurrence— assuming that one is interested in the belief itself and does not regard it simply as a "symptom" or expression of something else that is *more interesting*—must be sought along different lines.

The second error in regarding complex psychosocial behavior, consisting of communications about ourselves and the world about us, as mere symptoms of neurological functioning is *epistemological*. In other words, it is an error pertaining not to any mistakes in observation or reasoning, as such, but rather to the way in which we organize and express our knowledge. In the present case, the error lies in making a symmetrical dualism between mental and physical (or bodily) symptoms, a dualism which is merely a habit of speech and to which no known observations can be found to correspond. Let us see if this is so. In medical practice, when we speak of physical disturbances, we mean either signs (for example, a fever) or symptoms (for example, pain). We speak of mental symptoms, on the other hand, when we refer to a patient's *communications about himself, others, and the world about him.* He might state that he is Napoleon or that he is being persecuted by the Communists. These would be considered mental symptoms *only* if the observer believed that the patient was *not* Napoleon or that he was *not* being persecuted by the Communists. This makes it apparent that the statement that "X is a mental symptom" involves rendering a judgment. The judgment entails, moreover, a covert comparison or matching of the patient's ideas, concepts, or beliefs with those of the observer and the society in which they live. The notion of mental symptom is therefore inextricably tied to the *social* (including *ethical*) *context* in which it is made in much the same way as the notion of bodily symptom is tied to an *anatomical* and *genetic context* (Szasz, 1957a, 1957b).

To sum up what has been said thus far: I have tried to show that for those who regard mental symptoms as signs of brain disease, the concept of mental illness is unnecessary and misleading. For what they mean is that people so labeled suffer from diseases of the brain; and, if that is what they mean, it would seem better for the sake of clarity to say that and not something else.

MENTAL ILLNESS AS A NAME FOR PROBLEMS IN LIVING

The term "mental illness" is widely used to describe something which is very different than a disease of the brain. Many people today take it for granted that living is an arduous process. Its hardship for modern man, moreover, derives not so much from a struggle for biological survival as from the stresses and strains inherent in the social intercourse of complex human personalities. In this context, the notion of mental illness is used to identify or describe some feature of an individual's so-called personality. Mental illness—as a deformity of the personality, so to speak—is then regarded as the *cause* of the human disharmony. It is implicit in this view that social intercourse between people is regarded as something *inherently harmonious*, its disturbance being due solely to the presence of "mental illness" in many people. This is obviously fallacious reasoning, for it makes the abstraction "mental illness" into a *cause*, even though this abstraction was created in the first place to serve only as a shorthand expression for certain types of human behavior. It now becomes necessary to ask: "What kinds of behavior are regarded as indicative of mental illness, and by whom?"

The concept of illness, whether bodily or mental, implies *deviation from some clearly defined norm*. In the case of physical illness, the norm is the structural and functional integrity of the human body. Thus, although the desirability of physical health, as such, is an ethical value, what health *is* can be stated in anatomical and physiological terms. What is the norm deviation from which is regarded as mental illness? This question cannot be easily answered. But whatever this norm might be, we can be certain of only one thing: namely, that it is a norm that must be stated in terms of *psychosocial, ethical,* and *legal* concepts. For example, notions such as "excessive repression" or "acting out an unconscious impulse" illustrate the use of psychological concepts for judging (so-called) mental health and illness. The idea that chronic hostility, vengefulness, or divorce are indicative of mental illness would be illustrations of the use of ethical norms (that is, the desirability of love, kindness, and a stable marriage relationship). Finally, the widespread psychiatric opinion that only a mentally ill person would commit homicide illustrates the use of a legal concept as a norm of mental health. The norm from which deviation is measured whenever one speaks of a mental illness is a *psychosocial and ethical one*. Yet, the remedy is sought in terms of *medical* measures which—it is hoped and assumed—are free from wide differences of ethical value. The definition of the disorder and the terms in which its remedy are sought are therefore at serious odds with one another. The practical significance of this covert conflict between the alleged nature of the defect and the remedy can hardly be exaggerated.

Having identified the norms used to measure deviations in cases of mental illness, we will now turn to the question: "Who defines the norms and hence the deviation?" Two basic answers may be offered: (*a*) It may be the person himself (that is, the patient) who decides that he deviates from a norm. For example, an artist may believe that he suffers from a work inhibition; and he may implement this conclusion by seeking help *for* himself from a psychotherapist. (*b*) It may be someone other than the patient who decides that the latter is deviant (for example, relatives, physicians, legal authorities, society generally, etc.). In such a case a psychiatrist may be hired by others to do something *to* the patient in order to correct the deviation.

These considerations underscore the importance of asking the question "Whose agent is the psychiatrist?" and of giving a candid answer to it (Szasz, 1956, 1958). The psychiatrist (psychologist or nonmedical psychotherapist), it now develops, may be the agent of the patient, of the relatives, of the school, of the military services, of a business organization, of a court of law, and so forth. In speaking of the psychiatrist as the agent of these persons or organizations, it is not implied that his values concerning norms, or his ideas and aims concerning the proper nature of remedial action, need to coincide exactly with those of his employer. For example, a patient in individual psychotherapy may believe that his salvation lies in a new marriage; his psychotherapist need not share this hypothesis. As the patient's agent, however, he must abstain from bringing social or legal force to bear on the patient which would prevent him from putting his beliefs into action. If his *contract* is with the patient, the psychiatrist (psychotherapist) may disagree with him or stop his treatment; but he cannot engage others to obstruct the patient's aspirations. Similarly, if a psychiatrist is engaged by a court to determine the sanity of a criminal, he need not fully share the legal authorities' values and intentions in regard to the criminal and the means available for dealing with him. But the psychiatrist is expressly barred from stating, for example, that it is not the criminal who is "insane" but the men who wrote the law on the basis of which the very actions that are being judged are regarded as "criminal." Such an opinion could be voiced, of course, but not in a courtroom, and not by a psychiatrist who makes it his practice to assist the court in performing its daily work.

To recapitulate: In actual contemporary social usage, the finding of a mental illness is made by establishing a deviance in behavior from certain psychosocial, ethical, or legal norms. The judgment may be made, as in medicine, by the patient, the physician (psychiatrist), or others. Remedial action, finally, tends to be sought in a therapeutic—or covertly medical—framework, thus creating a situation in which *psychosocial, ethical,* and/or *legal deviations* are claimed to be correctible by (so-called) *medical action*. Since medical action is designed to correct only medical deviations, it seems logically absurd to expect that it will help solve problems whose very existence had been defined and established on nonmedical grounds. I think that these considerations may be fruitfully applied to the present use of tranquilizers and, more generally, to what might be expected of drugs of whatever type in regard to the amelioration or solution of problems in human living.

THE ROLE OF ETHICS IN PSYCHIATRY

Anything that people *do*—in contrast to things that *happen* to them (Peters, 1958)—takes place in a context of value. In this broad sense, no human activity is devoid of ethical implications. When the values underlying certain activities are widely shared, those who participate in their pursuit may lose sight of them altogether. The discipline of medicine, both as a pure science (for example, research) and as a technology (for example, therapy), contains many ethical considerations and judgments. Unfortunately, these are often denied, minimized, or merely kept out of focus; for the ideal of the medical profession as well as of the people whom it serves seems to be having a system of medicine (allegedly) free of ethical value. This sentimental notion is expressed by such things as the doctor's willingness to treat and help patients irrespective of their religious or political beliefs, whether they are rich or poor, etc. While there may be some grounds for this belief—albeit it is a view that is not impressively true even in these regards—the fact remains that ethical considerations encompass a vast range of human affairs. By making the practice of medicine neutral in regard to some specific issues of value need not, and cannot, mean that it can be kept free from all such values. The practice of medicine is intimately tied to ethics; and the first thing that we must do, it seems to me, is to try to make this clear and explicit. I shall let this matter rest here, for it does not concern us specifically in this essay. Lest there be any vagueness, however, about how or where ethics and medicine meet, let me remind the reader of such issues as birth control, abortion, suicide, and euthanasia as only a few of the major areas of current ethicomedical controversy.

Psychiatry, I submit, is very much more intimately tied to problems of ethics than is medicine. I use the word "psychiatry" here to refer to that contemporary discipline which is concerned with *problems in living* (and not with diseases of the brain, which are problems for neurology). Problems in human relations can be analyzed, interpreted, and given meaning only within given social and ethical contexts. Accordingly, it *does* make a difference—arguments to the contrary notwithstanding—what the psychiatrist's socioethical orientations happen to be; for these will influence his ideas on what is wrong with the patient, what deserves comment or interpretation, in what possible directions change might be desirable, and so forth. Even in medicine proper, these factors play a role, as for instance, in the divergent orientations which physicians, depending on their religious affiliations, have toward such things as birth control and therapeutic abortion. Can anyone really believe that a psychotherapist's ideas concerning religious belief, slavery, or other similar issues play no role in his practical work? If they do make a difference, what are we to infer from it? Does it not seem reasonable that we ought to have different psychiatric therapies—each expressly recognized for the ethical positions which they embody—for, say, Catholics and Jews, religious persons and agnostics, democrats and communists, white supremacists and Negroes, and so on? Indeed, if we look at how psychiatry is actually practiced today (especially in the United States), we find that people do seek psychiatric help in accordance with their social status and ethical beliefs (Hollingshead & Redlich, 1958). This should really not surprise us more than being told that practicing Catholics rarely frequent birth control clinics.

The foregoing position which holds that contemporary psychotherapists deal with problems in living, rather than with mental illnesses and their cures, stands in opposition to a currently prevalent claim, according to which mental illness is just as "real" and "objective" as bodily illness. This is a confusing claim since it is never known exactly what is meant by such words as "real" and "objective." I suspect, however, that what is intended by the proponents of this view is to create the idea in the popular mind that mental illness is some sort of disease entity, like an infection or a malignancy. If this were true, one could *catch* or *get* a "mental illness," one might *have* or *harbor* it, one might *transmit* it to others, and finally one could get *rid* of it. In my opinion, there is not a shred of evidence to support this idea. To the contrary, all the evidence is the other way and supports the view that what people now call mental illnesses are for the most part *communications* expressing unacceptable ideas, often framed, moreover, in an unusual idiom. The scope of this essay allows me to do no more than mention this alternative theoretical approach to this problem (Szasz, 1957c).

This is not the place to consider in detail the similarities and differences between bodily and mental illnesses. It shall suffice for us here to emphasize only one important difference between them: namely, that whereas bodily disease refers to public, physicochemical occurrences, the notion of mental illness is used to codify relatively more private, sociopsychological happenings of which the observer (diagnostician) forms a part. In other words, the psychiatrist does not stand *apart* from what he observes, but is, in Harry Stack Sullivan's apt words, a "participant observer." This means that he is *committed* to some picture of what he considers reality—and to what he thinks society considers reality—and he observes and judges the patient's behavior in the light of these considerations. This touches on our earlier observation that the notion of mental symptom itself implies a comparison between observer and observed, psychiatrist and patient. This is so obvious that I may be charged with belaboring trivialities. Let me therefore say once more that my aim in presenting this argument was expressly to criticize and counter a prevailing contemporary tendency to deny the moral aspects of psychiatry (and psychotherapy) and to substitute for them allegedly value-free medical considerations. Psychotherapy, for example, is being widely practiced as though it entailed nothing other than restoring the patient from a state of mental sickness to one of mental health. While it is generally accepted that mental illness has something to do with man's social (or interpersonal) relations, it is paradoxically maintained that problems of values (that is, of ethics) do not arise in this process.[1] Yet, in one sense, much of psychotherapy may revolve around nothing other than the elucidation and weighing of goals and values— many of which may be mutually contradictory—and the means whereby they might best be harmonized, realized, or relinquished.

The diversity of human values and the methods by means of which they may be realized is so vast, and many of them remain so unacknowledged, that they cannot fail but lead to conflicts in human relations. Indeed, to say that human relations at all levels—from mother to child, through husband and wife, to nation and nation—are fraught with stress, strain, and disharmony is, once again, making the obvious explicit. Yet, what may be obvious may be also poorly understood. This I think is the case here. For it seems to me that—at least in our scientific theories of behavior—we have failed to *accept* the simple fact that human relations are inherently fraught with difficulties and that to make them even relatively harmonious requires much patience and hard work. I submit that the idea of mental illness is now being put to work to obscure certain difficulties which at present may be inherent—not that they need be unmodifiable—in the social intercourse of persons. If this is true, the concept functions as a disguise; for instead of calling attention to conflicting human needs, aspirations, and values, the notion of mental illness provides an amoral and impersonal "thing" (an "illness") as an explanation for *problems in living* (Szasz, 1959). We may recall in this connection that not so long ago it was devils and witches who were held responsible for men's problems in social living. The belief in mental illness, as something other than man's trouble in getting along with his fellow man, is the proper heir to the belief in demonology and witchcraft. Mental illness exists or is "real" in exactly the same sense in which witches existed or were "real."

CHOICE, RESPONSIBILITY, AND PSYCHIATRY

While I have argued that mental illnesses do not exist, I obviously did not imply that the social and psychological occurrences to which this label is currently being attached also do not exist. Like the personal and social troubles which people had in the Middle Ages, they are real enough. It is the labels we give them that concerns us and, having labelled them, what we do about them. While I cannot go into the ramified implications of this problem here, it is worth noting that a demonologic conception of problems in living gave

rise to therapy along theological lines. Today, a belief in
mental illness implies—nay, requires—therapy along medical
or psychotherapeutic lines.

What is implied in the line of thought set forth here is
something quite different. I do not intend to offer a new conception of "psychiatric illness" nor a new form of "therapy."
My aim is more modest and yet also more ambitious. It is to
suggest that the phenomena now called mental illnesses be
looked at afresh and more simply, that they be removed from
the category of illnesses, and that they be regarded as the
expressions of man's struggle with the problem of *how* he
should live. The last mentioned problem is obviously a vast
one, its enormity reflecting not only man's inability to cope
with his environment, but even more his increasing self-
reflectiveness.

By problems in living, then, I refer to that truly explosive
chain reaction which began with man's fall from divine grace
by partaking of the fruit of the tree of knowledge. Man's
awareness of himself and of the world about him seems to be
a steadily expanding one, bringing in its wake an ever larger
burden of understanding (an expression borrowed from
Susanne Langer, 1953). *This burden, then, is to be expected
and must not be misinterpreted.* Our only *rational* means for
lightening it is *more understanding*, and appropriate *action*
based on such understanding. The main alternative lies in
acting as though the burden were not what in fact we perceive it to be and taking refuge in an outmoded theological
view of man. In the latter view, man does not fashion his life
and much of his world about him, but merely lives out his
fate in a world created by superior beings. This may logically
lead to pleading nonresponsibility in the face of seemingly
unfathomable problems and difficulties. Yet, if man fails to
take increasing responsibility for his actions, individually as
well as collectively, it seems unlikely that some higher power
or being would assume this task and carry this burden for
him. Moreover, this seems hardly the proper time in human
history for obscuring the issue of man's responsibility for his
actions by hiding it behind the skirt of an all-explaining conception of mental illness.

CONCLUSIONS

I have tried to show that the notion of mental illness has outlived whatever usefulness it might have had and that it now functions merely as a convenient myth. As such, it is a true heir to religious myths in general, and to the belief in witchcraft in particular; the role of all these belief-systems was to act as *social tranquilizers*, thus encouraging the hope that mastery of certain specific problems may be achieved by means of substitutive (symbolic-magical) operations. The notion of mental illness thus serves mainly to obscure the everyday fact that life for most people is a continuous struggle, not for biological survival, but for a "place in the sun," "peace of mind," or some other human value. For man aware of himself and of the world about him, once the needs for preserving the body (and perhaps the race) are more or less satisfied, the problem arises as to what he should do with himself. Sustained adherence to the myth of mental illness allows people to avoid facing this problem, believing that mental health, conceived as the absence of mental illness, automatically insures the making of right and safe choices in one's conduct of life. But the facts are all the other way. It is the making of good choices in life that others regard, retrospectively, as good mental health!

The myth of mental illness encourages us, moreover, to believe in its logical corollary: that social intercourse would be harmonious, satisfying, and the secure basis of a "good life" were it not for the disrupting influences of mental illness or "psychopathology." The potentiality for universal human happiness, in this form at least, seems to me but another example of the I-wish-it-were-true type of fantasy. I do believe that human happiness or well-being on a hitherto unimaginably large scale, and not just for a select few, is possible. This goal could be achieved, however, only at the cost of many men, and not just a few being willing and able to tackle their personal, social, and ethical conflicts. This means having the courage and integrity to forego waging battles on false fronts, finding solutions for substitute problems—for instance, fighting the battle of stomach acid and chronic fatigue instead of facing up to a marital conflict.

Our adversaries are not demons, witches, fate, or mental illness. We have no enemy whom we can fight, exorcise, or dispel by "cure." What we do have are *problems in living*— whether these be biologic, economic, political, or socio-psychological. In this essay I was concerned only with problems belonging in the last mentioned category, and within this group mainly with those pertaining to moral values. The field to which modern psychiatry addresses itself is vast, and I made no effort to encompass it all. My argument was limited to the proposition that mental illness is a myth, whose function it is to disguise and thus render more palatable the bitter pill of moral conflicts in human relations.

Personality Disorder *Is* Disease

DAVID P. AUSUBEL

In two recent articles in the *American Psychologist*, Szasz (1960) and Mowrer (1960) have argued the case for discarding the concept of mental illness. The essence of Mowrer's position is that since medical science lacks "demonstrated competence . . . in psychiatry," psychology would be wise to "get out" from "under the penumbra of medicine," and to regard the behavior disorders as manifestations of sin rather than of disease (p. 302). Szasz' position, as we shall see shortly, is somewhat more complex than Mowrer's, but agrees

FROM the *American Psychologist* 16 (1961) 69–74. Reprinted by permission of the author and publisher.

with the latter in emphasizing the moral as opposed to the psychopathological basis of abnormal behavior.

For a long time now, clinical psychology has both repudiated the relevance of moral judgment and accountability for assessing behavioral acts and choices, and has chafed under medical (psychiatric) control and authority in diagnosing and treating the personality disorders. One can readily appreciate, therefore, Mowrer's eagerness to sever the historical and professional ties that bind clinical psychology to medicine, even if this means denying that psychological disturbances constitute a form of illness, and even if psychology's close working relationship with psychiatry must be replaced by a new rapprochement with sin and theology, as "the lesser of two evils" (pp. 302–303). One can also sympathize with Mowrer's and Szasz' dissatisfaction with prevailing amoral and nonjudgmental trends in clinical psychology and with their entirely commendable efforts to restore moral judgment and accountability to a respectable place among the criteria used in evaluating human behavior, both normal and abnormal.

Opposition to these two trends in the handling of the behavior disorders (i.e., to medical control and to nonjudgmental therapeutic attitudes), however, does not necessarily imply abandonment of the concept of mental illness. There is no inconsistency whatsoever in maintaining, on the one hand, that most purposeful human activity has a moral aspect the reality of which psychologists cannot afford to ignore (Ausubel, 1952, p. 462), that man is morally accountable for the majority of his misdeeds (Ausubel, 1952, p. 469), and that psychological rather than medical training and sophistication are basic to competence in the personality disorders (Ausubel, 1956, p. 101), and affirming, on the other hand, that the latter disorders are genuine manifestations of illness. In recent years psychology has been steadily moving away from the formerly fashionable stance of ethical neutrality in the behavioral sciences; and in spite of strident medical claims regarding superior professional qualifications and preclusive legal responsibility for treating psychiatric patients, and notwithstanding the nominally restrictive provisions of medical practice acts, clinical psychologists have been assuming an increasingly more important, independent, and responsible role in treating the mentally ill population of the United States.

It would be instructive at this point to examine the tactics of certain other medically allied professions in freeing themselves from medical control and in acquiring independent, legally recognized professional status. In no instance have they resorted to the devious stratagem of denying that they were treating diseases, in the hope of mollifying medical opposition and legitimizing their own professional activities. They took the position instead that simply because a given condition is defined as a disease, its treatment need not necessarily be turned over to doctors of medicine if other equally competent professional specialists were available. That this position is legally and politically tenable is demonstrated by the fact that an impressively large number of recognized diseases are legally treated today by both medical *and* nonmedical specialists (e.g., diseases of the mouth, face, jaws, teeth, eyes, and feet). And there are few convincing reasons for believing that psychiatrists wield that much more political power than physicians, maxillofacial surgeons, ophthalmologists, and orthopedic surgeons, that they could be successful where these latter specialists have failed, in legally restricting practice in their particular area of competence to holders of the medical degree. Hence, even if psychologists were not currently managing to hold their own vis-à-vis psychiatrists, it would be far less dangerous and much more forthright to press for the necessary ameliorative legislation than to seek cover behind an outmoded and thoroughly discredited conception of the behavior disorders.

THE SZASZ-MOWRER POSITION

Szasz' (1960) contention that the concept of mental illness "now functions merely as a convenient myth" (p. 118) is grounded on four unsubstantiated and logically untenable propositions, which can be fairly summarized as follows:

1. Only symptoms resulting from demonstrable physical lesions qualify as legitimate manifestations of disease. Brain

pathology is a type of physical lesion, but its symptoms properly speaking, are neurological rather than psychological in nature. Under no circumstances, therefore, can mental symptoms be considered a form of illness.

2. A basic dichotomy exists between *mental* symptoms, on the one hand, which are subjective in nature, dependent on subjective judgment and personal involvement of the observer, and referable to cultural-ethical norms, and *physical* symptoms, on the other hand, which are allegedly objective in nature, ascertainable without personal involvement of the observer, and independent of cultural norms and ethical standards. Only symptoms possessing the latter set of characteristics are genuinely reflective of illness and amenable to medical treatment.

3. Mental symptoms are merely expressions of problems of living and, hence, cannot be regarded as manifestations of a pathological condition. The concept of mental illness is misleading and demonological because it seeks to explain psychological disturbance in particular and human disharmony in general in terms of a metaphorical but nonexistent disease entity, instead of attributing them to inherent difficulties in coming to grips with elusive problems of choice and responsibility.

4. Personality disorders, therefore, can be most fruitfully conceptualized as products of moral conflict, confusion, and aberration. Mowrer (1960) extends this latter proposition to include the dictum that psychiatric symptoms are primarily reflective of unacknowledged sin, and that individuals manifesting these symptoms are responsible for and deserve their suffering, both because of their original transgressions and because they refuse to avow and expiate their guilt (pp. 301, 304).

Widespread adoption of the Szasz-Mowrer view of the personality disorders would, in my opinion, turn back the psychiatric clock twenty-five hundred years. The most significant and perhaps the only real advance registered by mankind in evolving a rational and humane method of handling behavioral aberrations has been in substituting a concept of disease for the demonological and retributional doctrines regarding their nature and etiology that flourished until comparatively recent times. Conceptualized as illness, the symptoms of personality disorders can be interpreted in the light of underlying stresses and resistances, both genic and environmental, and can be evaluated in relation to *specifiable* quantitative and qualitative norms of appropriately adaptive behavior, both cross-culturally and within a particular cultural context. It would behoove us, therefore, before we abandon the concept of mental illness and return to the medieval doctrine of unexpiated sin or adopt Szasz' ambiguous criterion of difficulty in ethical choice and responsibility, to subject the foregoing propositions to careful and detailed study.

Mental Symptoms and Brain Pathology

Although I agree with Szasz in rejecting the doctrine that ultimately some neuroanatomic or neurophysiologic defect will be discovered in *all* cases of personality disorder, I disagree with his reasons for not accepting this proposition. Notwithstanding Szasz' straw man presentation of their position, the proponents of the extreme somatic view do not really assert that the *particular nature* of a patient's disordered beliefs can be correlated with "certain definite lesions in the nervous system" (Szasz, 1960, p. 113). They hold rather that normal cognitive and behavioral functioning depends on the anatomic and physiologic integrity of certain key areas of the brain, and that impairment of this substrate integrity, therefore, provides a physical basis for disturbed ideation and behavior, but does not explain, except in a very gross way, the particular kinds of symptoms involved. In fact, they are generally inclined to attribute the *specific* character of the patient's symptoms to the nature of his pre-illness personality structure, the substrate integrity of which is impaired by the lesion or metabolic defect in question.

Nevertheless, even though this type of reasoning plausibly accounts for the psychological symptoms found in general paresis, various toxic deleria, and other comparable conditions, it is an extremely improbable explanation of *all* instances of personality disorder. Unlike the tissues of any other organ, brain tissue possesses the unique property of making possible awareness of and adjustment to the world of sensory, social, and symbolic stimulation. Hence by virtue of this unique relationship of the nervous system to the environment, diseases of behavior and personality may reflect abnormalities in personal and social adjustment, quite apart from any structural or metabolic disturbance in the underlying neural substrate. I would conclude, therefore, that although brain pathology is probably not the most important cause of behavior disorder, it is undoubtedly responsible for the incidence of *some* psychological abnormalities *as well as* for various neurological signs and symptoms.

But even if we completely accepted Szasz' view that brain pathology does not account for any symptoms of personality disorder, it would still be unnecessary to accept his assertion that to qualify as a genuine manifestation of disease a given symptom must be caused by a physical lesion. Adoption of such a criterion would be arbitrary and inconsistent both with medical and lay connotations of the term "disease," which in current usage is generally regarded as including any marked deviation, physical, mental, or behavioral, from normally desirable standards of structural and functional integrity.

Mental versus Physical Symptoms

Szasz contends that since the analogy between physical and mental symptoms is patently fallacious, the postulated parallelism between physical and mental disease is logically untenable. This line of reasoning is based on the assumption that the two categories of symptoms can be sharply dichotomized with respect to such basic dimensions as objectivity-subjectivity, the relevance of cultural norms, and the need for personal involvement of the observer. In my opinion, the existence of such a dichotomy cannot be empirically demonstrated in convincing fashion.

Practically all symptoms of bodily disease involve some elements of subjective judgment—both on the part of the patient and of the physician. Pain is perhaps the most important and commonly used criterion of physical illness. Yet, any evaluation of its reported locus, intensity, character, and duration is dependent upon the patient's subjective appraisal of his own sensations and on the physician's assessment of the latter's pain threshold, intelligence, and personality structure. It is also a medical commonplace that the severity of pain in most instances of bodily illness may be mitigated by the administration of a placebo. Furthermore, in taking a meaningful history the physician must not only serve as a participant observer but also as a skilled interpreter of human behavior. It is the rare patient who does not react psychologically to the signs of physical illness; and hence physicians are constantly called upon to decide, for example, to what extent precordial pain and reported tightness in the chest are manifestations of coronary insufficiency, of fear of cardiac disease and impending death, or of combinations of both conditions. Even such allegedly objective signs as pulse rate, BMR, blood pressure, and blood cholesterol have their subjective and relativistic aspects. Pulse rate and blood pressure are notoriously susceptible to emotional influences, and BMR and blood cholesterol fluctuate widely from one cultural environment to another (Dreyfuss & Czaczkes, 1959). And anyone who believes that ethical norms have no relevance for physical illness has obviously failed to consider the problems confronting Catholic patients and/or physicians when issues of contraception, abortion, and preferential saving of the mother's as against the fetus' life must be faced in the context of various obstetrical emergencies and medical contraindications to pregnancy.

It should now be clear, therefore, that symptoms not only do not need a physical basis to qualify as manifestations of illness, but also that the evaluation of *all* symptoms, physical as well as mental, is dependent in large measure on subjective judgment, emotional factors, cultural-ethical norms, and personal involvement on the part of the observer. These considerations alone render no longer tenable Szasz' contention (1960, p. 114) that there is an inherent contradiction between using cultural and ethical norms as criteria of mental disease, on the one hand, and of employing medical measures of treatment on the other. But even if the postulated dichotomy between mental and physical symptoms were valid, the use of physical measures in treating subjective and relativistic psychological symptoms would still be warranted. Once we accept the proposition that impairment of the neutral substrate of personality can result in behavior disorder, it is logically consistent to accept the corollary proposition that other kinds of manipulation of the same neutral substrate can conceivably have therapeutic effects, irrespective of whether the underlying cause of the mental symptoms is physical or psychological.

Mental Illness and Problems of Living

. "The phenomena now called mental illness," argues Szasz (1960), can be regarded more forthrightly and simply as "expressions of man's struggle with the problem of how he should live" (p. 117). This statement undoubtedly oversimplifies the nature of personality disorders; but even if it were adequately inclusive it would not be inconsistent with the position that these disorders are a manifestation of illness. There is no valid reason why a particular symptom cannot both reflect a problem in living *and* constitute a manifestation of disease. The notion of mental illness, conceived in this way, would not "obscure the everyday fact that life for most people is a continuous struggle . . . for a 'place in the sun,' 'peace of mind,' or some other human value" (p. 118). It is quite true, as Szasz points out, that "human relations are inherently fraught with difficulties" (p. 117), and that most people manage to cope with such difficulties without becoming mentally ill. But conceding this fact hardly precludes the possibility that some individuals, either because of the magnitude of the stress involved, or because of genically or environmentally induced susceptibility to ordinary degrees of stress, respond to the problems of living with behavior that is either seriously distorted or sufficiently unadaptive to prevent normal interpersonal relations and vocational functioning. The latter outcome—gross deviation from a designated range of desirable behavioral variability— conforms to the generally understood meaning of mental illness.

The plausibility of subsuming abnormal behavioral reactions to stress under the general rubric of disease is further enhanced by the fact that these reactions include the same three principal categories of symptoms found in physical illness. Depression and catastrophic impairment of self-esteem, for example, are manifestations of personality disorder which are symptomologically comparable to edema in cardiac failure or to heart murmurs in valvular disease. They are indicative of underlying pathology but are neither adaptive nor adjustive. Symptoms such as hypomanic overactivity and compulsive striving toward unrealistically high achievement goals, on the other hand, are both adaptive and adjustive, and constitute a type of compensatory response to basic feelings of inadequacy, which is not unlike cardiac hypertrophy in hypertensive heart disease or elevated white blood cell count in acute infections. And finally, distortive psychological defenses that have some adjustive value but are generally maladaptive (e.g., phobias, delusions, autistic fantasies) are analogous to the pathological situation found in conditions like pneumonia, in which the excessive outpouring of serum and phagocytes in defensive response to pathogenic bacteria literally causes the patient to drown in his own fluids.

Within the context of this same general proposition, Szasz repudiates the concept of mental illness as demonological in nature, i.e., as the "true heir to religious myths in general and to the belief in witchcraft in particular" (p. 118) because it allegedly employs a reified abstraction ("a deformity of personality") to account in causal terms both for "human disharmony" and for symptoms of behavior disorder (p. 114). But again he appears to be demolishing a straw man. Modern students of personality disorder do not regard mental illness as a cause of human disharmony, but as a co-manifestation with it of inherent difficulties in personal adjustment and interpersonal relations; and in so far as I can accurately interpret the literature, psychopathologists do not conceive of mental illness as a cause of particular behavioral symptoms but as a generic term under which these symptoms can be subsumed.

Mental Illness and Moral Responsibility

Szasz' final reason for regarding mental illness as a myth is really a corollary of his previously considered more general proposition that mental symptoms are essentially reflective of problems of living and hence do not legitimately qualify as manifestations of disease. It focuses on difficulties of ethical choice and responsibility as the particular life problems most likely to be productive of personality disorder. Mowrer (1960) further extends this corollary by asserting that neurotic and psychotic individuals are responsible for their suffering (p. 301), and that unacknowledged and unexpiated sin, in turn, is the basic cause of this suffering (p. 304). As previously suggested, however, one can plausibly accept the proposition that psychiatrists and clinical psychologists have erred in trying to divorce behavioral evaluation from ethical considerations, in conducting psychotherapy in an amoral setting, and in confusing the psychological explanation of unethical behavior with absolution from accountability for same, *without* necessarily endorsing the view that personality disorders are basically a reflection of sin, and that victims of these disorders are less ill than responsible for their symptoms (Ausubel, 1952, pp. 392–397, 465–471).

In the first place, it is possible in most instances (although admittedly difficult in some) to distinguish quite unambiguously between mental illness and ordinary cases of immorality. The vast majority of persons who are guilty of moral lapses knowingly violate their own ethical precepts for expediential reasons—despite being volitionally capable at the time, both of choosing the more moral alternative and of exercising the necessary inhibitory control (Ausubel, 1952, pp. 465–471). Such persons, also, usually do not exhibit any signs of behavior disorder. At crucial choice points in facing the problems of living they simply choose the opportunistic instead of the moral alternative. They are not mentally ill, but they are clearly accountable for their misconduct. Hence, since personality disorder and immorality are neither coextensive nor mutually exclusive conditions, the concept of mental illness need not necessarily obscure the issue of moral accountability.

Second, guilt may be a contributory factor in behavior disorder, but is by no means the only or principal cause thereof. Feelings of guilt may give rise to anxiety and depression; but in the absence of catastrophic impairment of self-esteem induced by *other* factors, these symptoms tend to be transitory and peripheral in nature (Ausubel, 1952, pp. 362–363). Repression of guilt, is more a consequence than a cause of anxiety. Guilt is repressed in order to avoid the anxiety producing trauma to self-esteem that would otherwise result if it were acknowledged. Repression per se enters the causal picture in anxiety only secondarily—by obviating "the possibility of punishment, confession, expiation, and other guilt reduction mechanisms" (Ausubel, 1952, p. 456). Furthermore, in most types of personality disorder other than anxiety, depression, and various complications of anxiety such as phobias, obsessions, and compulsion, guilt feelings are either not particularly prominent (schizophrenic reactions), or are conspicuously absent (e.g., classical cases of inadequate or aggressive, antisocial psychopathy).

Third, it is just as unreasonable to hold an individual responsible for symptoms of behavior disorder as to deem him accountable for symptoms of physical illness. He is no more culpable for his inability to cope with sociopsychological stress than he would be for his inability to resist the spread of infectious organisms. In those instances where warranted guilt feelings *do* contribute to personality disorder, the patient is accountable for the misdeeds underlying his guilt, but is hardly responsible for the symptoms brought on by the guilt feelings or for unlawful acts committed during his illness. Acknowledgment of guilt may be therapeutically beneficial under these circumstances, but punishment for the original misconduct should obviously be deferred until after recovery.

Lastly, even if it were true that all personality disorder is a reflection of sin and that people are accountable for their behavioral symptoms, it would still be unnecessary to deny that these symptoms are manifestations of disease. Illness is no less real because the victim happens to be culpable for his illness. A glutton with hypertensive heart disease undoubtedly aggravates his condition by overeating, and is culpable in part for the often fatal symptoms of his disease, but what reasonable person would claim that for this reason he is not really ill?

CONCLUSIONS

Four propositions in support of the argument for discarding the concept of mental illness were carefully examined, and the following conclusions were reached:

First, although brain pathology is probably not the major cause of personality disorder, it does account for *some* psychological symptoms by impairing the neural substrate of personality. In any case, however, a symptom need not reflect a physical lesion in order to qualify as a genuine manifestation of disease.

Second, Szasz' postulated dichotomy between mental and physical symptoms is untenable because the assessment of *all* symptoms is dependent to some extent on subjective judgment, emotional factors, cultural-ethical norms, and personal involvement of the observer. Furthermore, the use of medical measures in treating behavior disorders—irrespective of whether the underlying causes are neural or psychological—is defensible on the grounds that if inadvertent impairment of the neural substrate of personality can have distortive effects on behavior, directed manipulation of the same substrate may have therapeutic effects.

Third, there is no inherent contradiction in regarding mental symptoms both as expressions of problems in living *and* as manifestations of illness. The latter situation results when individuals are for various reasons unable to cope with such problems, and react with seriously distorted or maladaptive behavior. The three principal categories of behavioral symptoms—manifestations of impaired functioning, adaptive compensation, and defensive overreaction—are also found in bodily disease. The concept of mental illness has never been advanced as a demonological cause of human disharmony, but only as a co-manifestation with it of certain inescapable difficulties and hazards in personal and social adjustment. The same concept is also generally accepted as a generic term for all behavioral symptoms rather than as a reified cause of these symptoms.

Fourth, the view that personality disorder is less a manifestation of illness than of sin, i.e., of culpable inadequacy in meeting problems of ethical choice and responsibility, and that victims of behavior disorder are therefore morally accountable for their symptoms, is neither logically nor empirically tenable. In most instances immoral behavior and mental illness are clearly distinguishable conditions. Guilt is only a secondary etiological factor in anxiety and depression, and in other personality disorders is either not prominent or conspicuously absent. The issue of culpability for symptoms is largely irrelevant in handling the behavior disorders, and in any case does not detract from the reality of the illness.

In general, it is both unnecessary and potentially dangerous to discard the concept of mental illness on the grounds that only in this way can clinical psychology escape from the professional domination of medicine. Dentists, podiatrists, optometrists, and osteopaths have managed to acquire an independent professional status without rejecting the concept of disease. It is equally unnecessary and dangerous to substitute the doctrine of sin for illness in order to counteract prevailing amoral and nonjudgmental trends in psychotherapy. The hypothesis of repressed guilt does not adequately explain most kinds and instances of personality disorder, and the concept of mental illness does not preclude judgments of moral accountability where warranted. Definition of behavior disorder in terms of sin or of difficulties associated with ethical choice and responsibility would substitute theological disputation and philosophical wrangling about values for specifiable quantitative and qualitative criteria of disease.

Normal Deviants

ERVING GOFFMAN

Movement of the hospitalized patient as well as his subsequent movement into and within the community, is
affected by his status as a deviant member of society and the
stigma which is attached to this status. These characteristics
can be analyzed in abstraction from the intrinsic characteristics of his illness, although it is, of course, recognized that,
concretely, mental illnesses distinguish such patients from
other types of deviants. However, the problems that mental
patients face in adapting to hospital life, and the ex-mental
patients face in adapting to life outside the hospital, are ones
we can learn considerably about from available studies of
other groupings that meet with problematic social acceptance.

The individual in our society—as in any other—is socialized through a diffuse and continuing process into making
certain demands upon himself and certain demands for himself upon others. It is partly through the satisfaction of these
demands that the individual constructs an identity or self-
conception and cements it with self-esteem.

For some individuals, however, a realization occurs,
whether suddenly or gradually, that they are less or will be
treated as less than they have learned to expect of and for
themselves, and that the frustration of these ingrained
expectations is due to the possession of an attribute that
functions as a social stigma. Defining themselves as persons
who will run in a particular race, they come to find that they

FROM *The Patient and the Mental Hospital*, Milton Greenblatt, et al
(Editors), The Free Press, New York, 1957, 507–510. Reprinted by permission of the author and the publisher.

have been partly disqualified and involuntarily re-identified in terms of their disqualification. The new category to which they find they belong separates them from those whom they thought they were like, and brings them together with those from whom they previously differed. Often this realization is brought home in some institution such as a jail, hospital, or orphanage, where they learn a great deal about their stigma while in prolonged intimate contact with those who will be their fellow-sufferers. And very often face-to-face interaction with those who are not stigmatized will officially proceed on the assumption that the stigma is not real or relevant, and unofficially proceed on the assumption that it is or may at any time become so.

Our society appears to have several basic types of stigma. There are "tribal" stigmas, arising from unapproved racial, national, and religious affiliations. There are the stigmas attached to physical handicap, including—to stretch the term—those associated with the undesirable characteristics of female sex and old age. And there are stigmas pertaining to what is somehow seen as a decay of moral responsibility, involving those persons who are unemployed or who have a known record of alcoholism, addiction, sexual deviation, penal servitude, or who have been committed to a mental hospital.

Persons who have frustrated identity expectations because of a stigma find themselves "in a spot," and adapt to their situation in certain patterned ways. In this regard, there are interesting differences within and between each type of stigma. For example, tribal stigmas commonly incorporate whole kinships, tending to reinforce family solidarity, while physical stigmas tend to cut across the nuclear family, creating a special set of problems in this regard and ensuring that stigmatized groupings need not give rise to stigmatized groups. Nonetheless, there appear to be significant social processes common to all stigmatized groupings.

It is assumed here that a great deal of what is common to stigmatized people can and should be understood by making two kinds of conceptual simplifications; one is that these people are of the same culture as those who stigmatize them, and the other is that they are and remain psychologically normal. This is the sense of the term "normal deviant" to refer to these people. (The term "native minorities" might do as well except that it implies corporate features that are not always found.) One is led to make these two assumptions of normalcy, abstractly, because quite disparate stigmas give rise to similar social processes, and because persons "incorrectly" rejected tend to manifest the processes while those who are "incorrectly" accepted do not.

There are, of course, groupings of persons who are not socially accepted in certain ways and who are appreciably abnormal in one or both of the senses mentioned. The selves these people are denied are likely then to be ones to which they are not currently attached. (This is the case with true "Ghetto communities.") For such groupings, a different framework of analysis must be applied. But in the United States today, it appears that almost every type of unaccepted person can profitably be understood, *initially at least,* by separating his responses into two components—the part that can be understood without having to posit cultural or psychological deviation, and the part that cannot. If we sift out first what can be understood by assuming cultural and psychological normalcy, then what remains will be easier to understand and easier to subject to required but perhaps quite different frames of references. For example, one framework of analysis is necessary if we define the mental hospital as a place where people know they can "get away" with certain kinds of symptomatic behavior; another framework is necessary if we are to define that hospital as the place where an individual is assured certain kinds of acceptance as an ordinary person, even though his symptoms brand him as an extraordinary one. Similarly, a paranoid patient can place himself in two kinds of difficulty: Unless he is careful (he feels) those who are chasing him will catch him—a problem that requires psychiatric understanding whether he appreciates this or not; unless he conceals or resolves his paranoia, a part of him may know that he is not likely to get out of the hospital—and this places him in a spot that is not psychiatric at all, but rather similar to the convict's when he tells the parole board of his future plans.

The set of social processes—the social dynamics—common to normal deviants may be suggested under four headings:

1. *Intrapersonal:* This includes such phenomena as self-hate, dissociation and denial, "secondary gains," etc.

2. *Interpersonal responses within the deviant groupings:* Here one finds such things as the focusing of conversational interest upon one's deviancy, upon the plight of one's deviant grouping, upon atrocity stories illustrating the injustice of the wider society, upon fellow-deviants who have become heroes of participation in the wider society; the use of a "line" or "sad tale" to account for one's membership; the use toward one's own people of epithets and derogatory labels usually applied by hostile nondeviants; the tendency to internal ranking, leading to distantiation from one's extremely deviant brethren, etc.

3. *Interpersonal responses between members of the deviant grouping and the wider society:* This includes such phenomena as so-called oversensitivity to slights; concern lest one's innocent actions be taken as a sign of deviation; uncertainty as to whether others are perceiving one as a deviant, and as to what their "real" attitude is to deviants; vacillation between submissive withdrawal and aggressive assertiveness; identification of certain nondeviants as friends of one's people before whom it is possible to relax; total and differential "passing," and the concomitant problems; development of strategies through which to make known one's deviancy and yet put others at ease with it, etc.

4. *Collective responses:* Here would be considered such organized and deputized actions as formal discussion of mutual problems; staged satirical skits ironically expressing the views of the wider society; publication of partisan newspapers and magazines, dealing with the virtues of one's grouping and the injustices of society; formation of group leadership and a *cadre* of paid professionals who engage in lobbying and other pressure group activity; participation in intergroup games and civic ceremonials. It may be noted that these collective actions are often taken through voluntary associations formed by and for deviants, which provide also for mutual support and protected sociability, and that in

America, clubs for ex-mental patients have not so far proven very successful.

All of these processes can be found to be operative in varying degrees among patients in mental hospitals. It is suggested, therefore, that research utilizing this frame of reference would be useful in adding to our knowledge and understanding of relations between mental patients and the extra-hospital world. Ultimately, it should also contribute to discovery of ways to diminish the barriers that surround mental patients and to increase the flow and movement of patients more directly in accordance with their true potential for rehabilitation.

Paranoia and the Dynamics of Exclusion

EDWIN M. LEMERT

One of the few generalizations about psychotic behavior which sociologists have been able to make with a modicum of agreement and assurance is that such behavior is a result or manifestation of a disorder in communication between the individual and society. The generalization, of course, is a

FROM *Sociometry* 25 (1962) 2–20. Reprinted by permission of the author and the publisher.

The research for this paper was in part supported by a grant from the California State Department of Mental Hygiene, arranged with the assistance of Dr. W. A. Oliver, Associate Superintendent of Napa State Hospital, who also helped as a critical consultant and made the facilities of the hospital available.

large one, and, while it can be illustrated easily with case history materials, the need for its conceptual refinement and detailing of the process by which disruption of communication occurs in the dynamics of mental disorder has for some time been apparent. Among the more carefully reasoned attacks upon this problem is Cameron's formulation of the paranoid pseudocommunity (1).

In essence, the conception of the paranoid pseudocommunity can be stated as follows:

Paranoid persons are those whose inadequate social learning leads them in situations of unusual stress to incompetent social reactions. Out of the fragments of the social behavior of others the paranoid person symbolically organizes a pseudocommunity whose functions he perceives as focused on him. His reactions to this *supposed community* of response which he sees loaded with threat to himself bring him into open conflict with the actual community and lead to his temporary or permanent isolation from its affairs. The "real" community, which is unable to share in his attitudes and reactions, takes action through forcible restraint or retaliation *after* the paranoid person "bursts into defensive or vengeful activity" (1).

That the community to which the paranoid reacts is "pseudo" or without existential reality is made unequivocal by Cameron when he says:

As he (the paranoid person) begins attributing to others the attitudes which he has towards himself, he unintentionally organizes these others into a functional community, a group unified in their supposed reactions, attitudes and plans with respect to him. He in this way organizes individuals, some of whom are actual persons and some only inferred or imagined, into a whole which satisfies for the time being his immediate need for explanation but which brings no assurance with it, and usually serves to increase his tensions. The community he forms not only fails to correspond to any organization shared by others but actually contradicts this consensus. More than this, the actions ascribed by him to its personnel are not actually performed or maintained by them; *they are united in no common undertaking against him* (1). (Italics ours.)

The general insightfulness of Cameron's analysis cannot be gainsaid and the usefulness of some of his concepts is easily granted. Yet a serious question must be raised, based upon empirical inquiry, as to whether in actuality the insidious qualities of the community to which the paranoid reacts are pseudo or a symbolic fabrication. There is an alternative point of view, which is the burden of this paper, namely that, while the paranoid person reacts differentially to his social environment, it is also true that "others" react differentially to him and this reaction commonly if not typically involves covertly organized action and conspiratorial behavior in a very real sense. A further extension of our thesis is that these differential reactions are reciprocals of one another, being interwoven and concatenated at each and all phases of a process of exclusion which arises in a special kind of relationship. Delusions and associated behavior must be understood in a context of exclusion which attenuates this relationship and disrupts communication.

By thus shifting the clinical spotlight away from the individual to a relationship and a process, we make an explicit break with the conception of paranoia as a disease, a state, a condition, or a syndrome of symptoms. Furthermore, we find it unnecessary to postulate trauma of early childhood or arrested psychosexual development to account for the main features of paranoia—although we grant that these and other factors may condition its expression.

This conception of paranoia is neither simple *a priori* theory nor is it a proprietary product of sociology. There is a substantial body of writings and empirical researches in psychiatry and psychology which question the sufficiency of the individual as primary datum for the study of paranoia. Tyhurst, for example, concludes from his survey of this literature that reliance upon intrapsychic mechanisms and the "isolated organism" have been among the chief obstacles to fruitful discoveries about this disorder (18). Significantly, as Milner points out, the more complete the investigation of the cases the more frequently do unendurable external circumstances make their appearance (13). More precisely, a number of studies have ended with the conclusions that external circumstances—changes in norms and values, displacement, strange environments, isolation, and linguistic separation— may create a paranoid disposition in the absence of any special character structure (15). The recognition of paranoid reactions in elderly persons, alcoholics, and the deaf adds to the data generally consistent with our thesis. The finding that displaced persons who withstood a high degree of stress during war and captivity subsequently developed paranoid reactions when they were isolated in a foreign environment commands special attention among data requiring explanation in other than organic or psychodynamic terms (7, 10).

From what has been said thus far, it should be clear that our formulation and analysis will deal primarily with what Tyhurst (18) calls paranoid patterns of behavior rather than with a clinical entity in the classical Kraepelinian sense. Paranoid reactions, paranoid states, paranoid personality disturbances, as well as the seldom-diagnosed "true paranoia," which are found superimposed or associated with a wide variety of individual behavior or "symptoms," all provide a body of data for study so long as they assume priority over other behavior in meaningful social interaction. The elements of behavior upon which paranoid diagnoses are based—delusions, hostility, aggressiveness, suspicion, envy, stubbornness, jealousy, and ideas of reference—are readily comprehended and to some extent empathized by others as social reactions, in contrast to the bizarre, manneristic behavior of schizophrenia or the tempo and affect changes stressed in manic-depressive diagnoses. It is for this reason that paranoia suggests, more than any other forms of mental disorder, the possibility of fruitful sociological analysis.

DATA AND PROCEDURE

The first tentative conclusions which are presented here were drawn from a study of factors influencing decisions to commit mentally disordered persons to hospitals, undertaken with the cooperation of the Los Angeles County Department of Health in 1952. This included interviews by means of schedules with members of 44 families in Los Angeles County who were active petitioners in commitment proceedings and the study of 35 case records of public health officer commitments. In 16 of the former cases and in 7 of the latter, paranoid symptoms were conspicuously present. In these cases family members and others had plainly accepted or "normalized" paranoid behavior, in some instances longstanding, until other kinds of behavior or exigencies led to critical judgments that "there was something wrong" with the person in question, and, later, that hospitalization was necessary. Furthermore, these critical judgments seemed to signal changes in the family attitudes and behavior towards the affected persons which could be interpreted as contributing in different ways to the form and intensity of the paranoid symptoms.

In 1958 a more refined and hypothesis-directed study was made of eight cases of persons with prominent paranoid characteristics. Four of these had been admitted to the state hospital at Napa, California, where they were diagnosed as paranoid schizophrenic. Two other cases were located and investigated with the assistance of the district attorney in Martinez, California. One of the persons had previously been committed to a California state hospital, and the other had been held on an insanity petition but was freed after a jury trial. Added to these was one so-called "White House case," which had involved threats to a President of the United States, resulting in the person's commitment to St. Elizabeth's Hospital in Washington, D.C. A final case was that of a professional person with a history of chronic job difficulties, who was designated and regarded by his associates as "brash," "queer," "irritating," "hypercritical," and "thoroughly unlikeable."

In a very rough way the cases made up a continuum ranging from one with very elaborate delusions, through those in which fact and misinterpretation were difficult to separate, down to the last case, which comes closer to what some would call paranoid personality disturbance. A requirement for the selection of the cases was that there be no history or evidence of hallucinations and also that the persons be intellectually unimpaired. Seven of the cases were of males, five of whom were over 40 years of age. Three of the persons had been involved in repeated litigations. One man published a small, independent paper devoted to exposures of psychiatry and mental hospitals. Five of the men had been or were associated with organizations, as follows: a small-town high school, a government research bureau, an association of agricultural producers, a university, and a contracting business.

The investigation of the cases were as exhaustive as it was possible to make them, reaching relatives, work associates, employers, attorneys, police, physicians, public officials and any others who played significant roles in the lives of the persons involved. As many as 200 hours each were given to collecting data on some of the cases. Written materials, legal documents, publications and psychiatric histories were studied in addition to the interview data. Our procedure in the large was to adopt an interactional perspective which sensitized us to sociologically relevant behavior underlying or associated with the more apparent and formal contexts of mental disorder. In particular we were concerned to establish the order in which delusions and social exclusion occur and to determine whether exclusion takes conspiratorial form.

THE RELEVANT BEHAVIOR

In another paper (8) we have shown that psychotic symptoms as described in formal psychiatry are not relevant bases for predictions about changes in social status and social participation of persons in whom they appear. Apathy, hallucinations, hyperactivity, mood swings, tics, tremors, functional paralysis or tachychardias have no intrinsic social meanings. By the same token, neither do such imputed attributes as "lack of insight," "social incompetence," or "defective role-taking ability" favored by some sociologists as generic starting points for the analysis of mental disorders. Rather, it is behavior which puts strain on social relationships that leads to status changes: informal or formal exclusion from groups, definition as a "crank," or adjudication as insane and commitment to a mental hospital (8). This is true even where the grandiose and highly bizarre delusions of paranoia are present. Definition of the socially stressful aspects of this disorder is a minimum essential, if we are to account for its frequent occurrence in partially compensated or benign form in society, as well as account for its more familiar presence as an official psychiatric problem in a hospital setting.

It is necessary, however, to go beyond these elementary observations to make it pre-eminently clear that strain is an emergent product of a relationship in which the behaviors of two or more persons are relevant factors, and in which the strain is felt both by ego and *alter* or *alters*. The paranoid relationship includes reciprocating behaviors with attached emotions and meanings which, to be fully understood, must be described cubistically from at least two of its perspectives. On one hand the behavior of the individual must be seen from the perspective of others or that of a group, and conversely the behavior of others must be seen from the perspective of the involved individual.

From the vantage of others the individual in the paranoid relationship shows:

1.   A disregard for the values and norms of the primary group, revealed by giving priority to verbally definable values over those which are implicit, a lack of loyalty in return for confidences, and victimizing and intimidating persons in positions of weakness.

2.   A disregard for the implicit structure of groups, revealed by presuming to privileges not accorded him, and the threat or actual resort to formal means for achieving his goals.

The second items have a higher degree of relevancy than the first in an analysis of exclusion. Stated more simply, they mean that, to the group, the individual is an ambiguous figure whose behavior is uncertain, whose loyalty can't be counted on. In short, he is a person who can't be trusted because he threatens to expose informal power structures. This, we believe, is the essential reason for the frequently encountered idea that the paranoid person is "dangerous" (4).

If we adopt the perceptual set of ego and see others or groups through his eyes, the following aspects of their behavior become relevant:

1.   the spurious quality of the interaction between others and himself or between others interacting in his presence;

2. the overt avoidance of himself by others;
3. the structured exclusion of himself from interaction.

The items we have described thus far—playing fast and loose with the primary group values by the individual, and his exclusion from interaction—do not alone generate and maintain paranoia. It is additionally necessary that they emerge in an interdependent relationship which requires trust for its fulfillment. The relationship is a type in which the goals of the individual can be reached only through co-operation from particular others, and in which the ends held by others are realizable if cooperation is forthcoming from ego. This is deduced from the general proposition that co-operation rests upon perceived trust, which in turn is a function of communication (11). When communication is disrupted by exclusion, there is a lack of mutually perceived trust and the relationship becomes dilapidated or paranoid. We will now consider the process of exclusion by which this kind of relationship develops.

THE GENERIC PROCESS OF EXCLUSION

The paranoid process begins with persistent interpersonal difficulties between the individual and his family, or his work associates and superiors, or neighbors, or other persons in the community. These frequently or even typically arise out of bona fide or recognizable issues centering upon some actual or threatened loss of status for the individual. This is related to such things as the death of relatives, loss of a position, loss of professional certification, failure to be promoted, age and physiological life cycle changes, mutilations, and changes in family and marital relationships. The status changes are distinguished by the fact that they leave no alternative acceptable to the individual, from whence comes their "intolerable" or "unendurable" quality. For example: the man trained to be a teacher who loses his certificate, which means he can never teach; or the man of 50 years of age who is faced with loss of a promotion which is a regular order of upward mobility in an organization, who knows that he can't "start over"; or the wife undergoing hysterectomy, which mutilates her image as a woman.

In cases where no dramatic status loss can be discovered, a series of failures often is present, failures which may have been accepted or adjusted to, but with progressive tension as each new status situation is entered. The unendurability of the current status loss, which may appear unimportant to others, is a function of an intensified commitment, in some cases born of an awareness that there is a quota placed on failures in our society. Under some such circumstances, failures have followed the person, and his reputation as a "difficult person" has preceded him. This means that he often has the status of a stranger on trial in each new group he enters, and that the groups or organizations willing to take a chance on him are marginal from the standpoint of their probable tolerance for his actions.

The behavior of the individual—arrogance, insults, presumption of privilege and exploitation of weaknesses in others—initially has a segmental or checkered pattern in that it is confined to status-committing interactions. Outside of these, the person's behavior may be quite acceptable— courteous, considerate, kind, even indulgent. Likewise, other persons and members of groups vary considerably in their tolerance for the relevant behavior, depending on the extent to which it threatens individual and organizational values, impedes functions, or sets in motion embarrassing sequences of social actions. In the early generic period, tolerance by others for the individual's aggressive behavior generally speaking is broad, and it is very likely to be interpreted as a variation of normal behavior, particularly in the absence of biographical knowledge of the person. At most, people observe that "there is something odd about him," or "he must be upset," "or he is just ornery," or "I don't quite understand him" (3).

At some point in the chain of interactions, a new configuration takes place in perceptions others have of the individual, with shifts in figure-ground relations. The individual, as we have already indicated, is an ambiguous figure, comparable to textbook figures of stairs or outlined cubes which reverse themselves when studied intently. From a normal variant the person becomes "unreliable," "untrustworthy," "dangerous," or someone with whom others "do not wish to be involved." An illustration nicely apropos of this came out in the reaction of the head of a music department in a university when he granted an interview to a man who had worked for years on a theory to compose music mathematically:

> When he asked to be placed on the staff so that he could use the electronic computers of the University *I shifted my ground* . . . when I offered an objection to his theory, he became disturbed, so I changed my reaction to "yes and no."

As is clear from this, once the perceptual reorientation takes place, either as the outcome of continuous interaction or through the receipt of biographical information, interaction changes qualitatively. In our words it becomes *spurious*, distinguished by patronizing, evasion, "humoring," guiding conversation onto selected topics, underreaction, and silence, all calculated either to prevent intense interaction or to protect individual and group values by restricting access to them. When the interaction is between two or more persons in the individual's presence it is cued by a whole repertoire of subtle expressive signs which are meaningful only to them.

The net effects of spurious interaction are to:

1. stop the flow of information to ego;
2. create a discrepancy between expressed ideas and affect among those with whom he interacts;
3. make the situation or the group image an ambiguous one for ego, much as he is for others.

Needless to say this kind of spurious interaction is one of the most difficult for an adult in our society to cope with, because it complicates or makes decisions impossible for him and also because it is morally invidious.[2]

The process from inclusion to exclusion is by no means an even one. Both individuals and members of groups change their perceptions and reactions, and vacillation is common, depending upon the interplay of values, anxieties and guilt on both sides. Members of an excluding group may decide they have been unfair and seek to bring the individual back into their confidence. This overture may be rejected or used by ego as a means of further attack. We have also found that ego may capitulate, sometimes abjectly, to others and seek group re-entry, only to be rejected. In some cases compromises are struck and a partial reintegration of ego into informal social relations is achieved. The direction which informal exclusion takes depends upon ego's reactions, the degree of communication between his interactors, the composition and structure of the informal groups, and the perceptions of "key others" at points of interaction which directly affect ego's status.

ORGANIZATIONAL CRISIS AND FORMAL EXCLUSION

Thus far we have discussed exclusion as an informal process. Informal exclusion may take place but leave ego's formal status in an organization intact. So long as this status is preserved and rewards are sufficient to validate it on his terms, an uneasy peace between him and others may prevail. Yet ego's social isolation and his strong commitments make him an unpredictable factor; furthermore the rate of change and internal power struggles, especially in large and complex organizations, means that preconditions of stability may be short lived.

Organizational crises involving a paranoid relationship arise in several ways. The individual may act in ways which arouse intolerable anxieties in others, who demand that "something be done." Again, by going to higher authority or making appeals outside the organization, he may set in motion procedures which leave those in power no other choice than to take action. In some situations ego remains relatively quiescent and does not openly attack the organization. Action against him is set off by growing anxieties or calculated motives of associates—in some cases his immediate superiors. Finally, regular organizational procedures incidental to promotion, retirement or reassignment may precipitate the crisis.

Assuming a critical situation in which the conflict between the individual and members of the organization leads to action to formally exclude him, several possibilities exist. One is the transfer of ego from one department, branch or division of the organization to another, a device frequently resorted to in the armed services or in large corporations. This requires that the individual be persuaded to make the change and that some department will accept him. While this may be accomplished in different ways, not infrequently artifice, withholding information, bribery, or thinly disguised threats figure conspicuously among the means by which the transfer is brought about. Needless to say, there is a limit to which transfers can be employed as a solution to the problem, contingent upon the size of the organization and the previous diffusion of knowledge about the transferee.

Solution number two we call encapsulation, which, in brief, is a reorganization and redefinition of ego's status. This has the effect of isolating him from the organization and making him directly responsible to one or two superiors who act as his intermediators. The change is often made palatable to ego by enhancing some of the material rewards of his status. He may be nominally promoted or "kicked upstairs," given a larger office, or a separate secretary, or relieved of onerous duties. Sometimes a special status is created for him.

This type of solution often works because it is a kind of formal recognition by the organization of ego's intense commitment to his status and in part a victory for him over his enemies. It bypasses them and puts him into direct communication with higher authority who may communicate with him in a more direct manner. It also relieves his associates of further need to connive against him. This solution is sometimes used to dispose of troublesome corporation executives, high-ranking military officers, and academic *personae non gratae* in universities.

A third variety of solutions to the problem of paranoia in an organization is outright discharge, forced resignation or non-renewal of appointment. Finally, there may be an organized move to have the individual in the paranoid relationship placed on sick leave, or to compel him to take psychiatric treatment. The extreme expression of this is pressure (as on the family) or direct action to have the person committed to a mental hospital.

The order of the enumerated solutions to the paranoid problem in a rough way reflects the amount of risk associated with the alternatives, both as to the probabilities of failure and of damaging repercussions to the organization. Generally, organizations seem to show a good deal of resistance to making or carrying out decisions which require expulsion of the individual or forcing hospitalization, regardless of his mental condition. One reason for this is that the person may have power within the organization, based upon his position, or monopolized skills and information,[3] and unless there is a strong coalition against him the general conservatism of administrative judgments will run in his favor. Herman Wouk's novel of *The Caine Mutiny* dramatizes some of the difficulties of cashiering a person from a position of power in an essentially conservative military organization. An extreme of this conservatism is illustrated by one case in which we found a department head retained in his position in an organization even though he was actively hallucinating as well as expressing paranoid delusions.[4] Another factor working on the individual's side is that discharge of a person in a position of power reflects unfavorably upon those who placed him there. Ingroup solidarity of administrators may be involved, and the methods of the opposition may create sympathy for ego at higher levels.

Even when the person is almost totally excluded and informally isolated within an organization, he may have power outside. This weighs heavily when the external power can be invoked in some way, or when it automatically leads to raising questions as to the internal workings of the organization. This touches upon the more salient reason for reluctance to eject an uncooperative and retaliatory person, even when he is relatively unimportant to the organization. We refer to a kind of negative power derived from the vulnerability of organizations to unfavorable publicity and exposure of their private lives that are likely if the crisis proceeds to formal hearings, case review or litigation. This is an imminent possibility where paranoia exists. If hospital commitment is attempted, there is a possibility that a jury trial will be demanded, which will force leaders of the organization to defend their actions. If the crisis turns into a legal contest of this sort, it is not easy to prove insanity, and there may be damage suits. Even if the facts heavily support the petitioners, such contests can only throw unfavorable light upon the organization.

THE CONSPIRATORIAL NATURE
OF EXCLUSION

A conclusion from the foregoing is that organizational vulnerability as well as anticipations of retaliations from the paranoid person lay a functional basis for conspiracy among those seeking to contain or oust him. Probabilities are strong that a coalition will appear within the organization, integrated by a common commitment to oppose the paranoid person. This, the exclusionist group, demands loyalty, solidarity and secrecy from its members; it acts in accord with a common scheme and in varying degrees utilizes techniques of manipulation and misrepresentation.

Conspiracy in rudimentary form can be detected in informal exclusion apart from an organizational crisis. This was illustrated in an office research team in which staff members huddled around a water cooler to discuss the unwanted associate. They also used office telephones to arrange coffee breaks without him and employed symbolic cues in his presence, such as humming the Dragnet theme song when he approached the group. An office rule against extraneous conversation was introduced with the collusion of supervisors, ostensibly for everyone, actually to restrict the behavior of the isolated worker. In another case an interview schedule designed by a researcher was changed at a conference arranged without him. When he sought an explanation at a subsequent conference, his associates pretended to have no knowledge of the changes.

Conspiratorial behavior comes into sharpest focus during organizational crises in which the exclusionists who initiate action become an embattled group. There is a concerted effort to gain consensus for this view, to solidify the group and to halt close interaction with those unwilling to completely join the coalition. Efforts are also made to neutralize those who remain uncommitted but who can't be kept ignorant of the plans afoot. Thus an external appearance of unanimity is given even if it doesn't exist.

Much of the behavior of the group at this time is strategic in nature, with determined calculations as to "what we will do if he does this or that." In one of our cases, a member on a board of trustees spoke of the "game being played" with the person in controversy with them. Planned action may be carried to the length of agreeing upon the exact words to be used when confronted or challenged by the paranoid individual. Above all there is continuous, precise communication among exclusionists, exemplified in one case by mutual exchanging of copies of all letters sent and received from ego.

Concern about secrecy in such groups is revealed by such things as carefully closing doors and lowering of voices when ego is brought under discussion. Meeting places and times may be varied from normal procedures; documents may be filed in unusual places and certain telephones may not be used during a paranoid crisis.

The visibility of the individual's behavior is greatly magnified during this period; often he is the main topic of conversation among the exclusionists, while rumors of the difficulties spread to other groups, which in some cases may be drawn into the controversy. At a certain juncture steps are taken to keep the members of the ingroup continually informed of the individual's movements and, if possible, of his plans. In effect, if not in form, this amounts to spying. Members of one embattled group, for example, hired an outside person unknown to their accuser to take notes on a speech he delivered to enlist a community organization on his side. In another case, a person having an office opening onto that of a department head was persuaded to act as an informant for the nucleus of persons working to depose the head from his position of authority. This group also seriously debated placing an all-night watch in front of their perceived malefactor's house.

Concomitant with the magnified visibility of the paranoid individual come distortions of his image, most pronounced in the inner coterie of exclusionists. His size, physical strength, cunning, and anecdotes of his outrages are exaggerated, with a central thematic emphasis on the fact that he is dangerous. Some individuals give cause for such beliefs in that previously they have engaged in violence or threats, others do not. One encounters characteristic contradictions in interviews on this point, such as: "No, he has never struck anyone around here—just fought with the policemen at the State Capitol," or "No, I am not afraid of him, but one of these days he will explode."

It can be said parenthetically that the alleged dangerousness of paranoid persons storied in fiction and drama has never been systematically demonstrated. As a matter of fact, the only substantial data on this, from a study of delayed admissions, largely paranoid, to a mental hospital in Norway, disclosed that "neither the paranoiacs nor paranoids have been dangerous, and most not particularly troublesome" (14). Our interpretation of this, as suggested earlier, is that the imputed dangerousness of the paranoid individual does not come from physical fear but from the organizational threat he presents and the need to justify collective action against him.

However, this is not entirely tactical behavior—as is demonstrated by anxieties and tensions which mount among those in the coalition during the more critical phases of their interaction. Participants may develop fears quite analogous to those of classic conspirators. One leader in such a group spoke of the period of the paranoid crisis as a "week of terror," during which he was wracked with insomnia and "had to take his stomach pills." Projection was revealed by a trustee who, during a school crisis occasioned by discharge of an aggressive teacher, stated that he "watched his shadows," and "wondered if all would be well when he returned home at night." Such tensional states, working along with a kind of closure of communication within the group, are both a cause and an effect of amplified group interaction which distorts or symbolically rearranges the image of the person against whom they act.

Once the battle is won by the exclusionists, their version of the individual as dangerous becomes a crystallized rationale for official action. At this point misrepresentation becomes part of a more deliberate manipulation of ego. Gross misstatements, most frequently called "pretexts," become justifiable ways of getting his cooperation, for example, to get him to submit to psychiatric examination or detention preliminary to hospital commitment. This aspect of the process has been effectively detailed by Goffman, with his concept of a "betrayal funnel" through which a patient enters a hospital (5). We need not elaborate on this, other than to confirm its occurrence in the exclusion process, complicated in our cases by legal strictures and the ubiquitous risk of litigation.

THE GROWTH OF DELUSION

The general idea that the paranoid person symbolically fabricates the conspiracy against him is in our estimation incorrect or incomplete. Nor can we agree that he lacks insight, as is so frequently claimed. To the contrary, many paranoid persons properly realize that they are being isolated and excluded by concerted interaction, or that they are being manipulated. However, they are at a loss to estimate accurately or realistically the dimensions and form of the coalition arrayed against them.

As channels of communication are closed to the paranoid person, he has no means of getting feedback on consequences of his behavior, which is essential for correcting his interpretations of the social relationships and organization which he must rely on to define his status and give him identity. He can only read overt behavior without the informal context. Although he may properly infer that people are organized against him, he can only use confrontation or formal inquisitorial procedures to try to prove this. The paranoid person must provoke strong feelings in order to receive any kind of meaningful communication from others—hence his accusations, his bluntness, his insults. Ordinarily this is nondeliberate; nevertheless, in one complex case we found the person consciously provoking discussions to get readings from others on his behavior. This man said of himself: "Some people would describe me as very perceptive, others would describe me as very imperceptive."

The need for communication and the identity which goes

with it does a good deal to explain the preference of paranoid
persons for formal, legalistic, written communications, and
the care with which many of them preserve records of their
contracts with others. In some ways the resort to litigation
is best interpreted as the effort of the individual to compel
selected others to interact directly with him as equals, to
engineer a situation in which evasion is impossible. The fact
that the person is seldom satisfied with the outcome of his
letters, his petitions, complaints and writs testifies to their
function as devices for establishing contact and interaction
with others, as well as "setting the record straight." The wide
professional tolerance of lawyers for aggressive behavior in
court and the nature of Anglo-Saxon legal institutions, which
grew out of a revolt against conspiratorial or star-chamber
justice, mean that the individual will be heard. Furthermore
his charges must be answered; otherwise he wins by default.
Sometimes he wins small victories, even if he loses the big
ones. He may earn grudging respect as an adversary, and
sometimes shares a kind of legal camaraderie with others in
the courts. He gains an identity through notoriety.

REINFORCEMENT OF DELUSION

The accepted psychiatric view is that prognosis for paranoia is poor, that recoveries from "true" paranoia are rare,
with the implication that the individual's delusions more or
less express an unalterable pathological condition. Granting
that the individual's needs and dispositions and his self-
imposed isolation are significant factors in perpetuating his
delusional reactions, nevertheless there is an important social
context of delusions through which they are reinforced or
strengthened. This context is readily identifiable in the fixed
ideas and institutionalized procedures of protective, custodial,
and treatment organizations in our society. They stand out
in sharpest relief where paranoid persons have come into
contact with law enforcement agencies or have been hospitalized. The cumulative and interlocking impacts of such
agencies work strongly to nurture and sustain the massive

sense of injustice and need for identity which underlie the delusions and aggressive behavior of the paranoid individual.

Police in most communities have a well-defined concept of cranks, as they call them, although the exact criteria by which persons are so judged are not clear. Their patience is short with such persons: in some cases they investigate their original complaints and if they conclude that the person in question is a crank they tend to ignore him thereafter. His letters may be thrown away unanswered, or phone calls answered with patronizing reassurance or vague promises to take steps which never materialize.

Like the police, offices of district attorneys are frequently forced to deal with persons they refer to as cranks or soreheads. Some offices delegate a special deputy to handle these cases, quaintly referred to in one office as the "insane deputy." Some deputies say they can spot letters of cranks immediately, which means that they are unanswered or discarded. However, family or neighborhood quarrels offer almost insoluble difficulties in this respect, because often it is impossible to determine which of two parties is delusional. In one office some complainants are called "fifty-fifty," which is jargon meaning that it is impossible to say whether they are mentally stable. If one person seems to be persistently causing trouble, deputies may threaten to have him investigated, which, however, is seldom if ever done.

Both police and district attorney staffs operate continuously in situations in which their actions can have damaging legal or political repercussions. They tend to be tightly ingrouped and their initial reaction to outsiders or strangers is one of suspicion or distrust until they are proved harmless or friendly. Many of their office procedures and general manner reflect this—such as carefully recording in a log book names, time, and reason for calling of those who seek official interviews. In some instances a complainant is actually investigated before any business will be transacted with him.

When the paranoid person goes beyond local police and courts to seek redress through appeals to state or national authorities, he may meet with polite evasion, perfunctory treatment of his case or formalized distrust. Letters to administrative people may beget replies up to a certain point, but thereafter they are ignored. If letters to a highly placed authority carry threats, they may lead to an investigation by security agencies, motivated by the knowledge that assassinations are not unknown in American life. Sometimes redress is sought in legislatures, where private bills may be introduced, bills which by their nature can only be empty gestures.

In general, the contacts which the delusional person makes with formal organizations frequently disclose the same elements of shallow response, evasion or distrust which played a part in the generic process of exclusion. They become part of a selective or selected pattern of interaction which creates a social environment of uncertainty and ambiguity for the individual. They do little to correct and much to confirm his suspicion, distrust and delusional interpretations. Moreover, even the environment of treatment agencies may contribute to the furtherance of paranoid delusion, as Stanton and Schwartz have shown in their comments on communication within the mental hospital. They speak pointedly of the "pathology of communication" brought about by staff practices of ignoring explicit meanings in statements or actions of patients and reacting to inferred or imputed meanings, thereby creating a type of environment in which "the paranoid feels quite at home" (17).

Some paranoid or paranoid-like persons become well known locally or even throughout larger areas to some organizations. Persons and groups in the community are found to assume a characteristic stance towards such people—a stance of expectancy and preparedness. In one such case, police continually checked the whereabouts of the man and, when the governor came to speak on the courthouse steps, two officers were assigned the special task of watching the man as he stood in the crowd. Later, whenever he went to the state capitol, a number of state police were delegated to accompany him when he attended committee hearings or sought interviews with state officials.[5] The notoriety this man acquired because of his reputed great strength in tossing officers around like tenpins was an obvious source of pleasure to him, despite the implications of distrust conveyed by their presence.

It is arguable that occupying the role of the mistrusted person becomes a way of life for these paranoids, providing them with an identity not otherwise possible. Their volatile contentions with public officials, their issuance of writings, publications, litigations in *persona propria*, their overriding tendency to contest issues which other people dismiss as unimportant or as "too much bother" become a central theme for their lives, without which they would probably deteriorate.

If paranoia becomes a way of life for some people, it is also true that the difficult person with grandiose and persecutory ideas may fulfill certain marginal functions in organizations and communities. One is his scapegoat function, being made the subject of humorous by-play or conjectural gossip as people "wonder what he will be up to next." In his scapegoat role, the person may help integrate primary groups within larger organizations by directing aggressions and blame towards him and thus strengthening feelings of homogeneity and consensus of group members.

There are also instances in which the broad, grapeshot charges and accusations of the paranoid person function to articulate dissatisfactions of those who fear openly to criticize the leadership of the community, organization, or state, or of the informal power structures within these. Sometimes the paranoid person is the only one who openly espouses values of inarticulate and politically unrepresented segments of the population (12). The "plots" which attract the paranoid person's attention—dope rings, international communism, monopolistic "interests," popery, Jewry, or "psycho-politicians"—often reflect the vague and ill-formed fears and concerns of peripheral groups, which tend to validate his self-chosen role as a "protector." At times in organizational power plays and community conflicts his role may even be put to canny use by more representative groups as a means of embarrassing their opposition.

THE LARGER SOCIO-CULTURAL CONTEXT

Our comments draw to a close on the same polemic note with which they were begun, namely, that members of communities and organizations do unite in common effort against the paranoid person prior to or apart from any vindictive behavior on his part. The paranoid community is real rather than pseudo in that it is composed of reciprocal relationships and processes whose net results are informal and formal exclusion and attenuated communication.

The dynamics of exclusion of the paranoid person are made understandable in larger perspective by recognizing that decision making in American social organization is carried out in small, informal groups through casual and often subtle male interaction. Entree into such groups is ordinarily treated as a privilege rather than a right, and this privilege tends to be jealously guarded. Crucial decisions, including those to eject persons or to reorganize their status in larger formal organizations, are made secretly. The legal concept of "privileged communication" in part is a formal recognition of the necessity for making secret decisions within organizations.

Added to this is the emphasis placed upon conformity in our organization-oriented society and the growing tendency of organization elites to rely upon direct power for their purposes. This is commonly exercised to isolate and neutralize groups and individuals who oppose their policies both inside and outside of the organization. Formal structures may be manipulated or deliberately reorganized so that resistant groups and individuals are denied or removed from access to power or the available means to promote their deviant goals and values. One of the most readily effective ways of doing this is to interrupt, delay, or stop the flow of information.

It is the necessity to rationalize and justify such procedures on a democratic basis which leads to concealment of certain actions, misrepresentation of their underlying meaning, and even the resort to unethical or illegal means. The difficulty of securing sociological knowledge about these techniques, which we might call the "controls behind the controls," and the denials by those who use them that they exist are logical consequences of the perceived threat such knowledge and admissions become to informal power structures. The epiphenomena of power thus become a kind of shadowy world of our culture, inviting conjecture and condemnation.

CONCLUDING COMMENT

We have been concerned with a process of social exclusion and with the ways in which it contributes to the development of paranoid patterns of behavior. While the data emphasize the organizational forms of exclusion, we nevertheless believe that these are expressions of a generic process whose correlates will emerge from the study of paranoia in the family and other groups. The differential responses of the individual to the exigencies of organized exclusion are significant in the development of paranoid reactions only insofar as they partially determine the "intolerable" or "unendurable" quality of the status changes confronting him. Idiosyncratic life history factors of the sort stressed in more conventional psychiatric analyses may be involved, but equally important in our estimation are those which inhere in the status changes themselves, age being one of the more salient of these. In either case, once situational intolerability appears, the stage is set for the interactional process we have described.

Our cases, it will be noted, were all people who remained undeteriorated, in contact with others and carrying on militant activities oriented towards recognizable social values and institutions. Generalized suspiciousness in public places and unprovoked aggression against strangers were absent from their experiences. These facts, plus the relative absence of "true paranoia" among mental-hospital populations, leads us to conclude that the "pseudo-community" associated with random aggression (in Cameron's sense) is a sequel rather than an integral part of paranoid patterns. They are likely products of deterioration and fragmentation of personality appearing, when and if they do, in the paranoid person after long or intense periods of stress and complete social isolation.

Notes on the Sociology of Deviance

It is general practice in sociology to regard deviant behavior as an alien element in society. Deviance is considered a vagrant form of human activity, moving outside the more orderly currents of social life. And since this type of aberration could only occur (in theory) if something were wrong within the social organization itself, deviant behavior is described almost as if it were leakage from machinery in poor condition: it is an accidental result of disorder and anomie, a symptom of internal breakdown.

The purpose of the following remarks will be to review this conventional outlook and to argue that it provides too narrow a framework for the study of deviant behavior. Deviation, we will suggest, recalling Durkheim's classic statement on the subject, can often be understood as a normal product of stable institutions, a vital resource which is guarded and preserved by forces found in all human organizations.[1]

I

According to current theory, deviant behavior is most likely to occur when the sanctions governing conduct in any given setting seem to be contradictory.[2] This would be the case, for example, if the work rules posted by a company required one course of action from its employees and the longer-range policies of the company required quite another. Any situation marked by this kind of ambiguity, of course, can pose a

FROM *Social Problems* 9 (Spring, 1962) 307–314. Reprinted by permission of the author and the publisher.

serious dilemma for the individual: if he is careful to observe one set of demands imposed upon him, he runs the immediate risk of violating some other, and thus may find himself caught in a deviant stance no matter how earnestly he tries to avoid it. In this limited sense, deviance can be regarded a "normal" human response to "abnormal" social conditions, and the sociologist is therefore invited to assume that some sort of pathology exists within the social structure whenever deviant behavior makes an appearance.

This general approach is clearly more concerned with the *etiology* of deviant behavior than with its continuing social *history*—and as a result it often draws sociological attention away from an important area of inquiry. It may be safe to assume that naive acts of deviance, such as first criminal offenses, are provoked by strains in the local situation. But this is only the beginning of a much longer story, for deviant activities can generate a good deal of momentum once they are set into motion: they develop forms of organization, persist over time, and sometimes remain intact long after the strains which originally produced them have disappeared. In this respect, deviant activities are often absorbed into the main tissue of society and derive support from the same forces which stabilize other forms of social life. There are persons in society, for example, who make career commitments to deviant styles of conduct, impelled by some inner need for continuity rather than by any urgencies in the immediate social setting. There are groups in society which actively encourage new deviant trends, often prolonging them beyond the point where they represent an adaption to strain. These sources of support for deviant behavior are difficult to visualize when we use terms like "strain," "anomie," or "breakdown" in discussions of the problem. Such terms may help us explain how the social structure creates fresh deviant potential, but they do not help us explain how that potential is later shaped into durable, persisting social pattern.[3] The individual's need for self continuity and the group's offer of support are altogether normal processes, even if they are sometimes found in deviant situations; and thus the study of deviant behavior is as much a study of social organization as it is a study of *dis*organization and anomie.

II

From a sociological standpoint, deviance can be defined as conduct which is generally thought to require the attention of social control agencies—that is, conduct about which "something should be done." Deviance is not a property *inherent in* certain forms of behavior; it is a property *conferred upon* these forms by the audiences which directly or indirectly witness them. Sociologically, then, the critical variable in the study of deviance is the social *audience* rather than the individual *person*, since it is the audience which eventually decides whether or not any given action or actions will become a visible case of deviation.

This definition may seem a little indirect, but it has the advantage of bringing a neglected sociological issue into proper focus. When a community acts to control the behavior of one of its members, it is engaged in a very intricate process of selection. Even a determined miscreant conforms in most of his daily behavior—using the correct spoon at mealtime, taking good care of his mother, or otherwise observing the mores of his society—and if the community elects to bring sanctions against him for the occasions when he does act offensively, it is responding to a few deviant details set within a vast context of proper conduct. Thus a person may be jailed or hospitalized for a few scattered moments of misbehavior, defined as a full-time deviant despite the fact that he had supplied the community with countless other indications that he was a decent, moral citizen. The screening device which sifts these telling details out of the individual's over-all performance, then, is a sensitive instrument of social control. It is important to note that this screen takes a number of factors into account which are not directly related to the deviant act itself: it is concerned with the actor's social class, his past record as an offender, the amount of remorse he manages to convey, and many similar concerns which take hold in the shifting moods of the community. This is why the community often overlooks behavior which seems technically deviant (like certain kinds of white collar graft) or takes sharp exception to behavior which seems essentially harmless (like certain kinds of sexual impropriety). It is an easily demonstrated fact, for example, that working class boys who steal cars are far more likely to go to prison than upper class boys who commit the same or even more serious crimes, suggesting that from the point of view of the community lower class offenders are somehow more deviant. To this extent, the community screen is perhaps a more relevant subject for sociological research than the actual behavior which is filtered through it.

Once the problem is phrased in this way, we can ask: how does a community decide what forms of conduct should be singled out for this kind of attention? And why, having made this choice, does it create special institutions to deal with the persons who enact them? The standard answer to this question is that society sets up the machinery of control in order to protect itself against the "harmful" effects of deviance, in much the same way that an organism mobilizes its resources to combat an invasion of germs. At times, however, this classroom convention only seems to make the problem more complicated. In the first place, as Durkheim pointed out some years ago, it is by no means clear that all acts considered deviant in a culture are in fact (or even in principle) harmful to group life.[4] And in the second place, specialists in crime and mental health have long suggested that deviance can play an important role in keeping the social order intact —again a point we owe originally to Durkheim.[5] This has serious implications for sociological theory in general.

III

In recent years, sociological theory has become more and more concerned with the concept "social system"—an organization of society's component parts into a form which sustains internal equilibrium, resists change, and is boundary maintaining. Now this concept has many abstract dimensions, but it is generally used to describe those forces in the social order which promote a high level of uniformity among human actors and a high degree of symmetry within human institutions. In this sense, the concept is normatively oriented since it directs the observer's attention toward those centers in social space where the core values of society are figuratively located. The main organizational principle of a system, then, is essentially a centripetal one: it draws the behavior of actors toward the nucleus of the system, bringing it within range of basic norms. Any conduct which is neither attracted toward this nerve center by the rewards of conformity nor compelled toward it by other social pressures is considered "out of control," which is to say, deviant.

This basic model has provided the theme for most contemporary thinking about deviance, and as a result little attention has been given to the notion that systems operate to maintain boundaries. Generally speaking, boundaries are controls which limit the fluctuation of a system's component parts so that the whole retains a defined range of activity— a unique pattern of constancy and stability—within the larger environment.[6] The range of human behavior is potentially so great that any *social* system must make clear statements about the nature and location of its boundaries, placing limits on the flow of behavior so that it circulates within a given cultural area. Thus boundaries are a crucial point of reference for persons living within any system, a prominent concept in the group's special language and tradition. A juvenile gang may define its boundaries by the amount of territory it defends, a professional society by the range of subjects it discusses, a fraternal order by the variety of members it accepts. But in each case, members share the same idea as to where the group begins and ends in social space and know what kinds of experience "belong" within this domain.

For all its apparent abstractness, a social system is organized around the movements of persons joined together in regular social relations. The only material found in a system for marking boundaries, then, is the behavior of its participants; and the form of behavior which best performs this function would seem to be deviant almost by definition, since it is the most extreme variety of conduct to be found within the experience of the group. In this respect, transactions taking place between deviant persons on the one side and agencies of control on the other are boundary maintaining mechanisms. They mark the outside limits of the area in which the norm has jurisdiction, and in this way assert how much diversity and variability can be contained within the system before it begins to lose its distinct structure, its unique shape.

A social norm is rarely expressed as a firm rule or official code. It is an abstract synthesis of the many separate times a community has stated its sentiments on a given issue. Thus the norm has a history much like that of an article of common law: it is an accumulation of decisions made by the community over a long period of time which gradually gathers enough moral influence to serve as a precedent for future decisions. Like an article of common law, the norm retains its validity only if it is regularly used as a basis for judgment. Each time the community censures some act of deviance, then, it sharpens the authority of the violated norm and re-establishes the boundaries of the group.

One of the most interesting features of control institutions, in this regard, is the amount of publicity they have always attracted. In an earlier day, correction of deviant offenders took place in the public market and gave the crowd a chance to display its interest in a direct, active way. In our own day, the guilty are no longer paraded in public places, but instead we are confronted by a heavy flow of newspaper and radio reports which offer much the same kind of entertainment. Why are these reports considered "newsworthy" and why do they rate the extraordinary attention they receive? Perhaps they satisfy a number of psychological perversities among the mass audience, as many commentators have suggested, but at the same time they constitute our main source of information about the normative outlines of society. They are lessons through which we teach one another what the norms mean and how far they extend. In a figurative sense, at least, morality and immorality meet at the public scaffold, and it is during this meeting that the community declares where the line between them should be drawn.

Human groups need to regulate the routine affairs of everyday life, and to this end the norms provide an important focus for behavior. But human groups also need to describe and anticipate those areas of being which lie beyond the immediate borders of the group—the unseen dangers which in any culture and in any age seem to threaten the security of group life. The universal folklore depicting demons, devils, witches and evil spirits may be one way to give form to these otherwise formless dangers, but the visible deviant is another kind of reminder. As a trespasser against the norm, he represents those forces excluded by the group's boundaries: he informs us, as it were, what evil looks like, what shapes the devil can assume. In doing so, he shows us the difference between kinds of experience which belong within the group and kinds of experience which belong outside it.

Thus deviance cannot be dismissed as behavior which *disrupts* stability in society, but is itself, in controlled quantities, an important condition for *preserving* stability.

IV

This raises a serious theoretical question. If we grant that deviant behavior often performs a valuable service in society, can we then assume that society as a whole actively tries to promote this resource? Can we assume, in other words, that some kind of active recruitment process is going on to assure society of a steady volume of deviance? Sociology has not yet developed a conceptual language in which this sort of question can be discussed without a great deal of circularity, but one observation can be made which gives the question an interesting perspective—namely, that deviant activities often seem to derive support from the very agencies designed to suppress them. Indeed, the institutions devised by human society for guarding against deviance sometimes seem so poorly equipped for this task that we might well ask why this is considered their "real" function at all.

It is by now a thoroughly familiar argument that many of the institutions built to inhibit deviance actually operate in such a way as to perpetuate it. For one thing, prisons, hospitals, and other agencies of control provide aid and protection for large numbers of deviant persons. But beyond this, such institutions gather marginal people into tightly segregated groups, give them an opportunity to teach one another the skills and attitudes of a deviant career, and even drive them into using these skills by reinforcing their sense of alienation from the rest of society.[7] This process is found not only in the institutions which actually confine the deviant, but in the general community as well.

The community's decision to bring deviant sanctions against an individual is not a simple act of censure. It is a sharp rite of transition, at once moving him out of his normal position in society and transferring him into a distinct deviant role.[8] The ceremonies which accomplish this change of status, usually, have three related phases. They arrange a formal *confrontation* between the deviant suspect and representatives of his community (as in the criminal trial or psychiatric case conference); they announce some *judgment* about the nature of his deviancy (a "verdict" or "diagnosis," for example); and they perform an act of social *placement*, assigning him to a special deviant role (like that of "prisoner" or "patient") for some period of time. Such ceremonies tend to be events of wide public interest and ordinarily take place in a dramatic, ritualized setting.[9] Perhaps the most obvious example of a commitment ceremony is the criminal trial, with its elaborate ritual and formality, but more modest equivalents can be found almost anywhere that procedures are set up for judging whether or not someone is officially deviant.

An important feature of these ceremonies in our culture is that they are almost irreversible. Most provisional roles conferred by society—like those of the student or citizen soldier, for instance—include some kind of terminal ceremony to mark the individual's movement back out of the role once its temporary advantages have been exhausted. But the roles allotted to the deviant seldom make allowance for this type of passage. He is ushered into the special position by a decisive and dramatic ceremony, yet is retired from it with hardly a word of public notice. As a result, the deviant often returns home with no proper license to resume a normal life in the community. From a ritual point of view, nothing has happened to cancel out the stigmas imposed upon him by earlier commitment ceremonies: the original verdict or diagnosis is still formally in effect. Partly for this reason, the community is apt to place the returning deviant on some form of probation within the group, suspicious that he will return to deviant activity upon a moment's provocation.

A circularity is thus set into motion which has all the earmarks of a "self-fulfilling prophecy," to use Merton's fine phrase. On the one hand, it seems obvious that the apprehensions of the community help destroy whatever chances the deviant might otherwise have for a successful return to society. Yet, on the other hand, everyday experience seems to show that these apprehensions are altogether reasonable, for it is a well-known and highly publicized fact that most ex-convicts return to prison and that a large proportion of mental patients require additional treatment after once having been discharged. The community's feeling that deviant persons cannot change, then, may be based on a faulty premise, but it is repeated so frequently and with such conviction that it eventually creates the facts which "prove" it correct. If the returned deviant encounters this feeling of distrust often enough, it is understandable that he too may begin to wonder if the original verdict or diagnosis is still in effect—and respond to this uncertainty by resuming deviant activity. In some respects, this solution may be the only way for the individual and his community to agree what forms of behavior are appropriate for him.

Moreover, this prophecy is found in the official policies of even the most advanced agencies of control. Police departments could not operate with any real effectiveness if they did not regard ex-convicts as an almost permanent population of offenders, a constant pool of suspects. Nor could psychiatric clinics do a responsible job if they did not view former patients as a group unusually susceptible to mental illness. Thus the prophecy gains currency at many levels within the social order, not only in the poorly informed attitudes of the community at large, but in the best informed theories of most control agencies as well.

In one form or another, this problem has been known to Western culture for many hundreds of years, and this simple fact is a very important one for sociology. For if the culture has supported a steady flow of deviant behavior throughout long periods of historical evolution, then the rules which apply to any form of functionalist thinking would suggest that strong forces must be at work to keep this flow intact. This may not be reason enough to assert that deviant behavior is altogether "functional"—in any of the many senses of that term—but it should make us reluctant to assume that the agencies of control are somehow organized to prevent deviant acts from occurring or to "cure" deviant offenders of their misbehavior.[10]

This in turn might suggest that our present models of the social system, with their clear emphasis on harmony and symmetry in social relations, only do a partial job of representing reality. Perhaps two different (and often conflicting) currents are found within any well-functioning system: those forces which promote a high over-all degree of conformity among human actors, and those forces which encourage some degree of diversity so that actors can be deployed throughout social space to mark the system's boundaries. In such a scheme, deviant behavior would appear as a variation on normative themes, a vital form of activity which outlines the area within which social life as such takes place.

As Georg Simmel wrote some years ago:

An absolutely centripetal and harmonious group, a pure "unification," not only is empirically unreal, it could show no real life process. . . . Just as the universe needs "love and hate," that is, attractive and repulsive forces, in order to have any form at all, so society, too, in order to attain a determinate shape, needs some quantitative ratio of harmony and disharmony, of association and competition, of favorable and unfavorable tendencies. . . . Society as we know it, is the result of both categories of interaction, which thus both manifest themselves as wholly positive.[11]

v

In summary, two new lines of inquiry seem to be indicated by the argument presented above.

First, this paper attempts to focus our attention on an old but still vital sociological question: how does a social structure communicate its "needs" or impose its "patterns" on human actors? In the present case, how does a social structure enlist actors to engage in deviant activity? Ordinarily, the fact that deviant behavior is more common in some sectors of society than in others is explained by declaring that something called "anomie" or "disorganization" prevails at these sensitive spots. Deviance leaks out where the social machinery is defective; it occurs where the social structure *fails* to communicate its needs to human actors. But if we consider the possibility that deviant persons are responding to the same social forces that elicit conformity from others, then we are engaged in another order of inquiry altogether. Perhaps the stability of some social units is maintained only if juvenile offenders are recruited to balance an adult majority; perhaps some families can remain intact only if one of their members becomes a visible deviant or is committed to a hospital or prison. If this supposition proves to be a useful one, sociologists should be interested in discovering how a social unit manages to differentiate the roles of its members and how certain persons are "chosen" to play the more deviant parts.

Second, it is evident that cultures vary in the way they regulate traffic moving back and forth from their deviant boundaries. Perhaps we could begin with the hypothesis that the traffic pattern known in our own culture has a marked Puritan cast: a defined portion of the population, largely drawn from young adult groups and from the lower economic classes, is stabilized in deviant roles and generally expected to remain there for indefinite periods of time. To this extent, Puritan attitudes about predestination and reprobation would seem to have retained a significant place in modern criminal law and public opinion. In other areas of the world, however, different traffic patterns are known. There are societies in which deviance is considered a natural pursuit for the young, an activity which they can easily abandon when they move through defined ceremonies into adulthood. There are societies which give license to large groups of persons to engage in deviant behavior for certain seasons or on certain days of the year. And there are societies in which special groups are formed to act in ways "contrary" to the normal expectations of the culture. Each of these patterns regulates deviant traffic differently, yet all of them provide some institutionalized means for an actor to give up a deviant "career" without permanent stigma. The problem for sociological theory in general might be to learn whether or not these varying patterns are functionally equivalent in some meaningful sense; the problem for applied sociology might be to see if we have anything to learn from those cultures which permit re-entry into normal social life to persons who have spent a period of "service" on society's boundaries.

Notes

INTRODUCTION

[1] Norman Dain, *Concepts of Insanity in the United States, 1789–1865*, New Brunswick, N. J.: Rutgers University Press, 1964.

[2] Norman Cameron and Ann Magaret, *Behavior Pathology*, Boston: Houghton Mifflin, 1951.

[3] Harry Stack Sullivan, *The Interpersonal Theory of Psychiatry* (Helen S. Perry and Marry L. Gawel, Eds.) New York: W. W. Norton, 1953.

[4] Thomas S. Szasz, *The Myth of Mental Illness: Foundations of a Theory of Personal Conduct*, New York: Hoeber, 1961. (Szasz's original article, "The Myth of Mental Illness," is reprinted in this volume.)

[5] Edwin M. Lemert, *Social Pathology*, New York: McGraw-Hill, 1951; Erving Goffman, *Asylums*, Garden City, N. Y.: Doubleday-Anchor, 1961. (Lemert's "Paranoia and the Dynamics of Exclusion," and Goffman's "Normal Deviants" are reprinted in this volume.)

[6] Ohmer Milton, *Behavior Disorders: Perspectives and Trends*, New York: Lippincott, 1965.

[7] Lyle Saunders, *Cultural Difference and Medical Care*, New York: Russell Sage, 1954.

[8] *Milwaukee Journal*, May 27, 1962.

[9] Joint Commission on Mental Illness and Health, *Action for Mental Health*, New York: Basic Books, 1961.

[10] *The Capital-Times*, August 15, 1962. Madison, Wisconsin.

SOME FACTORS IN IDENTIFYING AND DEFINING
MENTAL ILLNESS
David Mechanic

[1] Hollingshead, A. B., and R. C. Redlich, *Social Class and Mental Illness* (New York: John Wiley & Sons, 1958); Myers, J. K., and B. H. Roberts, *Family and Class Dynamics in Mental Illness* (New York: John Wiley & Sons, 1959); Clausen, J. A., and Marion R. Yarrow, eds., "The Impact of Mental Illness on the Family," *Journal of Social Issues*, 11 (December, 1955); Cumming, Elaine, and John Cumming, *Closed Ranks* (Cambridge, Mass.: Harvard University Press, 1957).

For an excellent study of the relationship between social class status and mode of treatment received, see Myers, J. K., and L. Schaffer, "Social Stratification and Psychiatric Practice: A Study of an Outpatient Clinic," *American Sociological Review*, 19 (June, 1954), 307–310.

[2] For some reviews of the problems of definition, see Jahoda, Marie, *Current Concepts of Positive Mental Health* (New York: Basic Books, Inc., 1958); Redlich, F. C., "The Concept of Health in Psychiatry," in Leighton, A. H., J. Clausen, and R. Wilson, eds., *Explorations in Social*

306

306   NOTES

Psychiatry (New York: Basic Books, Inc., 1957); and Cumming and Cumming. *op. cit.*

3 In an interesting experimental study, Jones and deCharms found that the degree to which a confederate is seen as responsible for his behavior when he causes the group to fail is a definite factor in evaluating his dependability. If he causes the group to fail, but is viewed as lacking the necessary ability to perform the necessary task, he is less likely to be defined as "undependable" than if he is viewed as lacking motivation.

See Jones, E. E., and R. deCharms, "Changes in Social Perception as a Function of the Personal Relevance of Behavior," *Sociometry*, 20 (March, 1957), 75–85. Kingsley Davis also presents an argument similar to the one offered in the text of this paper. *See* Davis, K., *Human Society* (New York: Macmillan Co., 1958), Chap. 10.

4 Public health programs attempt, in some measure, to change the lay evaluation of what constitutes "mental illness." A study by Woodward, J. L., "Changing Ideas on Mental Illness and Its Treatment," *American Sociological Review*, 16 (August, 1951), 443–454, indicates that in at least one community persons are becoming more sensitive to what physicians regard as signs of "mental illness." However, more recently, Shirley Star, in the analysis of data from a National Opinion Research Center survey, points out that for most people "mental illness" is associated with violent, unpredictable behavior.

The Cummings, *op. cit.*, found that persons in the community they studied had fairly simple notions about "mental illness," and that they were relatively immune to the influence of an educational mental health program. In their book they attempt to analyze why this program failed.

As the public image of "mental illness" slowly changes to conform more closely to that held by the professional psychiatrist, predictability and the ability to take the role of the other may become less important in the evaluation made by lay persons.

R. T. LaPiere, in *The Freudian Ethic* (New York: Duell, Sloan & Pearce, Inc., 1959) argues that the therapeutic ethic has influenced many segments of social action and that the consequences are that deviant persons are absolved from responsibility for their actions regardless of the direction of deviancy and the abilities of the evaluators to understand the motivation for deviancy. From this, argues LaPiere, stems the ideology of permissive and nonpunishing prisons, therapeutic schools for delinquents, etc.

5 Lemert has pointed out that when an "ill" person deviates from role expectancies, his social visibility increases and others are constrained to respond accordingly to his behavior. In cases of violence and disorderly conduct, police action more often is taken. Where less violent behaviors occur—delusion, hallucinations, restlessness—if action is to be taken at all, it is likely to be taken by more primary associates. See Lemert, E., "Legal Commitment and Social Control," *Sociology and Research*, 30 (May–June, 1946), 370–378.

6 In this regard, Jones and deCharms, *op. cit.*, found that behavior

does not appear to have a constant meaning, and that the attribution of stable characteristics to behavior is dependent on the significance of the behavior for the perceiver's own value-maintenance or goal attainment.

7 In his research Clausen et al., *op. cit.*, reports large differences in the degrees to which primary group members are willing to support and tolerate persons displaying schizophrenic symptoms. For excellent general reviews of the sociological mental health literature, see Clausen, J. A., "The Sociology of Mental Health," in Merton, R. K., L. Broom, and L. S. Cottrell, Jr., eds., *Sociology Today* (New York: Basic Books, Inc., 1959), 485–508; and Clausen, J. A. *Sociology and the Field of Mental Health* (New York: Russell Sage Foundation, 1956).

8 From time to time, situations do occur where the social group uses the label "mental illness" as an excuse to rid itself of one of its members, if his presence or behavior is becoming annoying. This seems to occur relatively frequently with aged members in our society.

The absence of a strong familial feeling of responsibility to the aged often leads to hospitalization, especially in cases where the person makes more than the usual demands for care and attention. Often it becomes convenient for the family to view increasing demands as symptoms of "mental illness."

9 The data in this general area lead to difficult problems of interpretation. Clausen writes:

"To explain, in part, the differential distribution of rates of hospitalization found by Faris and Dunham, Owen suggested that mentally ill persons are perceived and dealt with differently in different settings. Thus far, no one has demonstrated that the areas of the city and segments of the population with the highest rates of hospitalization are characterized by a higher rate of recognition of mental illness than are other areas. Several studies suggest that, if anything, the reverse is true. There is substantial documentation, however, of the fact that the social status of the mentally ill person tends to influence the perception by his family and others of the nature of his problem, their modes of dealing with him prior to his entering medical-psychiatric channels, and the kinds of services offered to him by psychiatric clinics or hospitals." (*Sociology Today, op. cit.*, 494–495.)

The difficulties with the available data stem from the fact that important effects work at cross-purposes, and the studies, thus far, have not adequately controlled for these effects. One such factor is the varying toleration levels in the different kinds of communities reported by Eaton, J., and R. J. Weil, *Culture and Mental Disorders: A Comparative Study of the Hutterites and Other Populations* (New York: The Free Press, 1955). They report that the Hutterite culture, which seemingly had little mental illness, in fact, had prevalence rates similar to those found in other groups, but that in this culture mental illness was handled differently from the way it was handled among other groups.

Thus, while there may be lesser visibility in larger social structures,

group toleration or the ability to make use of the psychologically handicapped may be more limited. Further research is needed in this general
area, with a clearer delineation and control of visibility, tolerance, and
role variables.

10 In this respect, the data reported by Glass are especially interesting. See Glass, A. J., "Psychotherapy in the Combat Zone," in *Symposium on Stress* (Washington, D.C.: Army Medical Service Graduate
School, Walter Reed Army Medical Hospital, 1953). He reports that
when psychiatry casualties were evacuated to psychiatric facilities
during the North African and Sicilian campaigns, few patients were
salvaged for combat duty.

The psychiatrist usually assumed the patient was "ill" and "sought
to uncover basic emotional conflicts or attempted to relate current behavior and symptoms with past personality patterns," which seemingly
provided patients with "rational" reasons for their combat failure. Both
patient and therapist were often readily convinced that the limit of
combat endurance had been reached.

On the other hand, when patients were subsequently treated in the
combat zone with such interpersonal devices as suggestion, influence,
etc., a much higher percentage were returned to combat.

As Clausen points out, "maintaining ties with their outfits and preserving a conception of themselves as somehow being able to cope seem
to have given many men the strength to do exactly that. . . . A good deal
of research is needed to learn under what circumstances withholding
the label "mental illness" may lead to more effective coping than
would combining, labeling and therapy." (See Clausen, *Sociology
Today, op. cit.*, 503.)

Clausen's comments are especially interesting because we have some
evidence that during periods of stress—with increasing social, psychological, and physical demands—rates of psychotic breakdown increase.
However, if group solidarity is essential and group vulnerability is
high, the sick role is not easily accorded to persons with neurotic-type
symptoms, and considerable pressure is placed upon them to continue
in their social roles.

See Mechanic, D., "Illness and Social Disability: Some Problems in
Analysis," *Pacific Sociological Review*, 2 (Spring, 1959), 37–41; and
Schneider, D. M., "Social Dynamics of Physical Disability in Army
Basic Training," in Kluckhohn, C., H. A. Murray, and A. M. Schneider,
eds., *Personality in Nature, Society, and Culture, second edition* (New
York: Alfred A. Knopf, 1956), 386–392.

The observations by Groen, C., "Psychogenesis and Psychotherapy of
Ulcerative Colitis," *Psychosomatic Medicine*, 9 (May–June, 1947), 151–
174, that the ulcer symptoms of his patients disappeared during the
stress conditions of concentration camp life and often reappeared after
leaving the concentration camp, raises some interesting questions, as
W. Caudill has observed. *See* Caudill, W., *Effects of Social and Cultural
Systems in Reactions to Stress* (New York: Social Science Research
Council, 1958).

Whether the change during incarceration is a reaction to the change in the stressors, or is tied with shifts in the physiological, psychological, and social systems accompanying camp life, is a question for further and better-controlled research. Also, Groen's observations that the wives were providing their husbands with more emotional support than formerly is an important variable.

11 The data collected by Hollingshead and Redlich, *op. cit.*, indicate that members of the lower strata are most likely to take this path to treatment centers.

12 A similar argument has been presented by Goffman, E., "The Moral Career of the Mental Patient," *Psychiatry*, 22 (May, 1959), 123–142, and Erikson, K. T., "Patient Role and Social Uncertainty—a Dilemma of the Mentally Ill," in Cohen, Mabel B., ed., *Advances in Psychiatry* (New York: W. W. Norton Co., 1959), 102–123.

WHAT THE MASS MEDIA PRESENT
Jum C. Nunnally, Jr.

1 The content analysis was directed by Dr. Wilbur Schramm and Dr. Wilson Taylor.

2 The recordings were made available by Dr. Dallas Smythe.

3 The study was conducted by Dr. Wilbur Schramm.

REJECTION: A POSSIBLE CONSEQUENCE OF SEEKING HELP FOR MENTAL DISORDERS
Derek L. Phillips

1 Joint Commission on Mental Illness and Health, *Action for Mental Health*, New York: Science Editions, 1961, p. 69.

2 See, for example, John A. Clausen and Marian R. Yarrow, "Paths to the Mental Hospital," *The Journal of Social Issues*, 11 (November, 1955), pp. 25–32; Elaine and John Cumming, *Closed Ranks: An Experiment in Mental Health Education*. Cambridge: Harvard University Press, 1957; Bruce P. Dohrenwend, Viola W. Bernard, and Lawrence C. Kolb, "The Orientations of Leaders in an Urban Area Toward Problems of Mental Illness," *The American Journal of Psychiatry*, 118 (February, 1962), pp. 683–691; Howard E. Freeman and Ozzie G. Simmons, "Mental Patients in the Community," *American Sociological Review*, 23 (April, 1958), pp. 147–154; Gerald Gurin, Joseph Veroff, and Sheila Feld, *Americans View Their Mental Health*, New York: Basic Books, 1960; E. Gartly Jaco, *The Social Epidemiology of Mental Disorders*, New York: Russell Sage Foundation, 1960; Paul V. Lemkau and Guido M. Crocetti, "An Urban Population's Opinion and Knowledge about Mental Illness," *The American Journal of Psychiatry*, 118.

3 See Clausen and Yarrow, *op. cit.*; and Cumming and Cumming, *op. cit.*

4 Star, *op. cit.*

5 Elaine and John Cumming, "Affective Symbolism, Social Norms, and Mental Illness," *Psychiatry*, 19 (February, 1956), pp. 77-85.

6 Lemkau and Crocetti, *op. cit.*, p. 694.

7 Dohrenwend, Bernard, and Kolb, *op. cit.*, p. 685.

8 Cumming and Cumming, *Closed Ranks, op. cit.*, p. 102.

9 See, for example, Gurin et al. *op. cit.*

10 Dohrenwend et al. *op. cit.*; Gurin et al., *op. cit.*; Ramsey and Seipp, *op. cit.*; Woodward, *op. cit.*

11 Clausen and Yarrow, *op. cit.*; Cumming and Cumming, *op. cit.*; Frederick C. Redlich, "What the Citizen Knows About Psychiatry," *Mental Hygiene*, 34 (January, 1950), pp. 64-70; Star, *op. cit.* (February, 1962), pp. 692-700; Jum C. Nunnally, Jr., *Popular Conceptions of Mental Health*, New York: Holt, Rinehart and Winston, 1961; Glen V. Ramsey and Melita Seipp, "Public Opinions and Information Concerning Mental Health," *Journal of Clinical Psychology*, 4 (October, 1948), pp. 397-406; Charlotte Green Schwartz, "Perspectives on Deviance— Wives' Definitions of Their Husbands' Mental Illness," *Psychiatry*, 20 (August, 1957), pp. 275-291; Shirley Star, "The Place of Psychiatry in Popular Thinking," paper presented at the meeting of the American Association for Public Opinion Research, Washington, D.C., May 1957; Julian L. Woodward, "Changing Ideas on Mental Illness and Its Treatment," *American Sociological Review*, 16 (August, 1951), pp. 443-454.

12 Gurin et al. *op. cit.*, p. 307.

13 *Ibid.*, p. 400.

14 Kasper D. Naegele, "Clergymen, Teachers, and Psychiatrists: A Study in Roles and Socialization," *The Canadian Journal of Economic and Political Science*, 22 (February, 1956), p. 48.

15 Clausen and Yarrow, *op. cit.*, p. 63.

16 Jack K. Ewalt, intro., Marie Jahoda, *Current Concepts of Positive Mental Health*, New York: Basic Books, 1958, p. xi.

17 Charles Kadushin, "Individual Decisions to Undertake Psycho-therapy," *Administrative Science Quarterly*, 3 (December, 1958), p. 389.

Gurin et al. report that 25 per cent of their respondents who had problems but did not utilize help tried to solve the problems by themselves, *op. cit.*, pp. 350-351.

18 The sample was drawn from the address section of the Directory, with every 15th address marked for interview. The first address was drawn randomly from the first 15 entries; thereafter every 15th address was included until the total sample of 300 was obtained.

19 Twenty-eight of the households drawn in the original sample refused to be interviewed. In each of these cases, a substitution was made by selecting an address at random from the same street. Four of these substitutes refused to be interviewed, necessitating further substitution. Also requiring substitution were three addresses that could not be located and six wives of household heads who were divorced, separated, or widowed, rather than married. Selecting substitutes from the same neighborhood was done on the assumption that persons living

in the same neighborhood would resemble one another in certain important ways; they were more likely, than people living in different neighborhoods, to be of similar socio-economic status. Although the possibility of bias still exists, so few substitutions were necessary that, hopefully, the effect is minimal.

20 In a pre-test with a sample of 32 women and 28 men, no significant differences were found between the rejection rates of men and women.

21 Star, *op. cit.*

22 The normal person was described as follows: "Here is a description of a man. Imagine that he is a respectable person living in your neighborhood. He is happy and cheerful, has a good enough job and is fairly well satisfied with it. He is always busy and has quite a few friends who think he is easy to get along with most of the time. Within the next few months he plans to marry a nice young woman he is engaged to."

23 My purpose was to determine (a) whether the rejection of the mentally ill descriptions might in part be accounted for by individuals who rejected everyone regardless of behavior; and (b) whether the utilization of a help-source alone could influence rejection, or whether it was the "combination" of deviant behavior and the use of a help-source that led to rejection.

24 The advantages of including tests of different combinations of two or more variables within one experiment have been cited by several writers concerned with experimental design. For example, D. J. Finney, *The Theory of Experimental Design*, Chicago: The University of Chicago Press, 1960, p. 68, notes the following advantages: "(1) To broaden the basis of inferences relating to one factor by testing that factor under various conditions of others; (2) To assess the extent to which the effects of one factor are modified by the level of others; (3) To economize in experimental material by obtaining information on several factors without increasing the size of the experiment beyond what would be required for one or two factors alone."

25 For two excellent explanations of the Graeco-Latin Square design see Finney, *op. cit.*, and E. F. Lindquist, *Design of Experiments in Psychology and Education*, Boston: Houghton Mifflin, 1953.

26 In addition, to 50 per cent of the respondents, the paranoid, the depressed individual, and the "normal" person were presented as males, with the simple schizophrenic and the phobic-compulsive individual presented as females. The other half of the sample saw a reversed order—the simple schizophrenic and the compulsive individuals as males, and the paranoid, depressed, and "normal" persons as females. Since both the male case abstracts and the female case abstracts were rejected in accordance with the pattern shown in Table 1, they will not be discussed further in this paper. The findings for the *differences* in the *absolute* rejection of males and females exhibiting a given behavior and utilizing the same help-source will be the subject of a forthcoming paper.

27 The above order duplicates the order of "closeness" represented by

the scale. The items, however, were administered to each respondent in a random fashion.

28 *See*, for example, Lindquist, *op. cit.*, chs. 12 and 13.

29 Following Lindquist, neither orders nor interaction was found to be statistically significant at the .20 level. See Lindquist, *op. cit.*, pp. 273–281.

30 For details of the classification procedures, see pp. 82–88 of the author's doctoral dissertation, of which this research is a part: "Help-Sources and Rejection of the Mentally Ill," unpublished Ph.D. Dissertation, Yale University, 1962.

31 For details of the authoritarian scale see *ibid.*, p. 77.

32 The question was: "We've been talking about people with worries and problems. Have any of your close friends or relatives had any psychiatric treatment or gone to a hospital or professional person, or community agency, regarding emotional problems?" If the respondent answered in the affirmative, she was asked who this person was.

33 Attitude toward self-reliance was measured by the respondent's reaction to the following statement: "People should be expected to handle their own problems," with a choice of four responses—strongly agree, agree somewhat, disagree somewhat, and strongly disagree.

34 Because our primary interest is in the effect of help-source rather than behavior, rejection rates will hereafter be presented in combined form only.

35 Talcott Parsons, *The Social System*, New York: The Free Press, 1950, p. 437. Parsons states that ". . . the fourth closely related element [in the sick role] is the obligation—in proportion to the severity of the condition, of course—to seek *technically competent* help, namely in the most usual case, that of a physician and to *cooperate* with him in the process of trying to get well." He makes this point again in "Definitions of Health and Illness in the Light of American Values and Social Structure," in E. Gartly Jaco (ed.), *Patients, Physicians and Illness*, New York: The Free Press, 1958, pp. 165–187.

36 We might expect those with help-seeking friends to reject in the same pattern as those with help-seeking relatives. Although both groups of respondents have had experience with someone who sought help, those whose experience was with friends probably were not so involved in the other's welfare and therefore had less intimate a knowledge of the help-sources people consult for emotional problems.

37 This is not surprising in light of the generally low rejection of the "normal" person.

38 Only 9 per cent disagreed (either somewhat or strongly) with the statement about people handling their own problems. This finding lends support to the proposition that people in our society are expected to handle their own problems.

39 Again we ignore differences *among* the various groups of respondents. Our primary interest is in determining whether the relation between help-source and rejection is maintained *within* each group.

40 It should be recalled that the latter respondents also rejected persons not seeking help more than persons seeing a psychiatrist; the

findings with respect to experience with a help-seeking relative and non-adherence to the norm of self-reliance are not entirely similar.

[41] It would have been desirable to control for experience and attitude toward self-reliance simultaneously, but there were too few (13) respondents who reported experience with a help-seeking relative *and* did not adhere to the norm of self-reliance.

[42] The small number of respondents with a help-seeking relative (37), and the small number not adhering to the norm of self-reliance (28), make these findings, as well as their interpretation, highly tentative.

[43] David Mechanic and Edmund A. Volkart, "Stress, Illness, and the Sick Role," *American Sociological Review*, 26 (February, 1961), pp. 51–58.

[44] Jaco, *op. cit.*, points out that "If mental disease carries a stigma in a particular community, it is likely that many families will use extreme measures to conceal the fact that a member is mentally ill; even to the extent of preventing him from obtaining psychiatric treatment in that area." (p. 18)

[45] For an interesting presentation of cost and reward, see George C. Homans, *Social Behavior: Its Elementary Forms*, New York: Harcourt, Brace & World, 1961, ch. 5.

THE ILLUSION OF DUE PROCESS IN COMMITMENT
PROCEEDINGS
Luis Kutner

[1] For a further account of this case see Wille, *Why Refugee Asked for Ticket to Russia*, Daily News, March 29, 1962, p. 10, col. 1.

[2] The Illinois Mental Health Code [ILL. REV. STAT. ch. 91½ (1961)], adopted in 1951, has been praised by some commentators as being particularly well conceived. *See*, e.g., Ross, *Commitment of the Mentally Ill*, 57 MICH. L. REV. 945, 949 (1959).

[3] Although the Mental Health Clinic in Cook County is perhaps not typical of those throughout the state, it is by far the largest, contributing 50 percent of Illinois' total commitments in 1961.

Much of the following textual discussion with respect to practices of the Mental Health Clinic was obtained by the author in a personal interview with Thaddeus V. Adesko, Judge, County Court of Cook County.

[4] Wille, *Feud at Mental Health Clinic Over Civil Rights*, Chicago Daily News, March 30, 1962, p. 20, col. 6.

[5] Wille, *The Mental Health Clinic—Expressway to Asylum*, Chicago Daily News, March 26, 1962, p. 10, col. 4.

[6] Wille, *How to Humanize Mental Clinic*, Chicago Daily News, March 31, 1962, p. 19, col. 2.

[7] Social workers on the [Cook County Mental Health] clinic staff

say that they have been instructed not to tell patients that they have a right to a jury trial.

"Supervisors haven't put this in writing—but they let you know their feelings in guarded terms," said one girl.

"When it was discovered that I told a patient that he could have a jury trial, I was severely reprimanded and ordered to 'co-operate with the doctors.' I was reminded that we are not civil service employees. We can be fired at any time."

Patients who do request a jury trial are often told they will have to wait "months" in the clinic for the trial, the social workers say.

Wille, *Feud at Mental Clinic Over Civil Rights*, Chicago Daily News, March 30, 1962, p. 20, col. 6.

For an account of a clinic social worker who was actually dismissed for telling a patient of his right to counsel and a jury trial, *see* Chicago Daily News, July 25, 1962, p. 4, col. 3.

8 See, e.g., Sheean *v.* Holman, 6 N.J. Misc. 346, 141 Atl. 170 (Sup. Ct. 1928) (commitment papers signed by two physicians who had never examined patient); *In re* Wertz, 118 N.E.2d 188 (Ohio App. 1954) (failure to comply with the requirement that alleged-mentally-ill be given notice of hearing); Lindsay *v.* Woods, 27 S.W.2d 263, 264 (Tex. Civ. App. 1930) (alleged-mentally-ill woman held incommunicado in a sanitarium prior to sanity hearing).

9 A fair hearing on notice, the right to counsel, and the right to a jury trial are not mere "technicalities," but represent principles of justice in dealing with human rights which have evolved over the centuries.

SOCIAL CONDITIONS FOR RATIONALITY: HOW URBAN AND RURAL COURTS DEAL WITH THE MENTALLY ILL
Thomas J. Scheff

1 Karl Mannheim, *Man and Society in an Age of Reconstruction* (London: Routledge, 1935), 52–54.

2 The larger study on which this paper is based is described in "Legal and Medical Decision-making in the Hospitalization of the Mentally Ill: A Field Study." (in press). For a detailed description of the psychiatric screening procedures, see the author's "The Societal Reaction to Deviance: Ascriptive Elements in the Psychiatric Screening of Mental Patients," *Social Problems* 11 (1964) 401–413.

3 Similar findings are reported in Herbert J. Jaffe, "Civil Commitment of the Mentally Ill," *Pennsylvania Law Review*, 107 (March 1959), 668–85; John H. Hess and Herbert E. Thomas, "Incompetency to Stand Trial; Procedures, Results and Problems," paper presented at the 1962 convention of the American Psychiatric Association; Kutner, "The Illusion of Due Process" . . . reprinted in this volume; Mechanic, "Some Factors in Identifying and Defining Mental Illness," reprinted in this volume; Robert Ross Mezer and Paul D. Rheingold, "Mental

Incapacity and Incompetency: A Psycho-Legal Problem," *American Journal of Psychiatry*, 118 (1962), 827–31 (note particularly the comment on p. 829 regarding the presumption of incapacity).

4 For a review of epidemiological studies of mental disorder see Richard J. Plunkett and John E. Gordon, *Epidemiology and Mental Illness*. Most of these studies suggest that at any given point in time, psychiatrists find a substantial proportion of persons in normal populations to be "mentally ill." One interpretation of this finding is that much of the deviance detected in these studies is of short duration. For a further discussion of this question, see Thomas J. Scheff, "The Role of the Mentally Ill and the Dynamics of Mental Disorder: A Research Framework," *Sociometry* 26 (December 1963), 436–53.

5 For an assessment of the evidence regarding the effectiveness of electroshock, drugs, psychotherapy, and other psychiatric treatments, see H. J. Eysenck, *Handbook of Abnormal Psychology*, Basic Books, New York, 1961, Part III.

6 For examples from military psychiatry, *see* Albert J. Glass, "Psychotherapy in the Combat Zone," in *Symposium on Stress* (Washington, D.C.: Army Medical Service Graduate School, 1953), and B. L. Bushard, "The U.S. Army's Mental Hygiene Consultation Service," in Symposium on Preventive and Social Psychiatry, 15–17 (April 1957) Walter Reed Army Institute of Research, Washington, D.C., pp. 431–43. For a discussion of essentially the same problem in the context of a civilian mental hospital, cf. Erikson, "Patient Role and Social Uncertainty."

7 Hugh Allen Ross, "Commitment of the Mentally Ill: Problems of Law and Policy," *Michigan Law Review*, 57 (1959), 145–1018, p. 962.

8 Charles E. Ares, Ann Rankin, and Herbert Sturz, "The Manhattan Bail Project: An Interim Report on the Use of Pre-Trial Parole," *New York University Law Review*, 38 (January 1963), 67–95.

9 U.S. Senate Hearings, *Inquiry into Satellite and Missile Programs*, 1958, quoted in Merton J. Peck and Frederick M. Scherer, *The Weapons Acquisition Process: An Economic Analysis* (Boston: Harvard U. Press, 1962), p. 245.

PSYCHIATRIC AND SOCIAL ATTRIBUTES AS PREDICTORS OF CASE OUTCOME IN MENTAL HOSPITALIZATION

Simon Dinitz, Mark Lefton, Shirley Angrist, and Benjamin Pasamanick

1 Howard E. Freeman and Ozzie G. Simmons, "Mental Patients in the Community: Family Settings and Performance Levels," *American Sociological Review*, 23 (April, 1958), pp. 147–154.

2 George W. Brown, "Experiences of Discharged Chronic Schizophrenic Patients in Various Types of Living Groups," *Milbank Memorial Fund Quarterly*, 37 (April, 1959), pp. 105–131.

3 Thomas A. C. Rennie and Leo Srole, "Social Class Prevalence and

316 NOTES

Distribution of Psychosomatic Conditions in an Urban Population,"
Psychosomatic Medicine, 18 (November-December, 1956), pp. 1–21.

4 August B. Hollingshead and Frederick C. Redlich, *Social Class and
Mental Illness*, New York: Wiley, 1958.

5 Copies of the scales can be obtained from the Columbus Psychiatric
Institute and Hospital.

6 The mean scores for these categories are 142.3, 160.5 and 172.2
respectively and are significantly different from each other (CR's
< .01).

7 For a more complete report of these relationships *see* Benjamin
Pasamanick and Leonard Ristine, "Differential Assessment of Post-
Hospital Psychological Functioning: Evaluations by Psychiatrists and
Relatives," *American Journal of Psychiatry*, in press.

8 Simon Dinitz, Mark Lefton, Jon Simpson, Benjamin Pasamanick,
and Ralph Patterson, "The Ward Behavior of Psychiatric Patients."
Social Problems, 6 (Fall, 1958), pp. 107–115.

9 Howard E. Freeman and Ozzie G. Simmons, *op. cit.*; Howard E.
Freeman and Ozzie G. Simmons, "Wives, Mothers, and Posthospital
Performance Levels," *Social Forces*, 37 (December, 1958), pp. 153–159;
Ozzie G. Simmons and Howard E. Freeman, "Familial Expectations
and Posthospital Performance of Mental Patients," *Human Relations*,
12 (August, 1959), pp. 233–242.

THE ABBOTTS
R. D. Laing and A. Esterson

1 For reasons given in the introduction, we are limiting ourselves
very largely to the transactional phenomenology of these family situations. Clearly, here and in every other family, the material we present
is full of evidence of the struggle of each of the family members
against their own sexuality. Maya without doubt acts on her own
sexual experience, in particular by way of splitting, projection, denial,
and so on. Although it is beyond the self-imposed limitation of our
particular focus in this book to discuss these aspects, the reader should
not suppose that we wish to deny or to minimize the person's *action on
himself* (what psycho-analysts usually call defence mechanisms), particularly in respect of sexual feelings aroused towards family members,
that is, in respect of incest.

SOCIAL FACTORS INFLUENCING THE DEVELOPMENT AND
CONTAINMENT OF PSYCHIATRIC SYMPTOMS
Jules V. Coleman

1 Saslow, George and Peters, A. D. A Follow-Up Study of "Untreated"
Patients with Various Behavior Disorders. *Psychiat. Quart.*, 1956, Vol.
30, 238–302.

2 Frank, Jerome D. *Persuasion and Healing. A Comparative Study of Psychotherapy.* Schocken Books, New York, 1963.

3 Errera, Paul. A Sixteen Year Follow-Up of Schizophrenic Patients Seen in An Outpatient Clinic. *AMA Archives of Neurology and Psychiatry,* Vol. 78, pp. 84–88, July 1957.

4 Errera, Paul and Coleman, J. V. A Long-Term Follow-Up Study of Neurotic Phobic Patients in a Psychiatric Clinic. *Journal of Nervous & Mental Disease,* Vol. 136, March 1963.

5 Ernst, K. *Die Prognose Der Neurosen.* Springer Verlag, Berlin, 1959.

6 Srole, Leo, et al. *Mental Health in the Metropolis. The Midtown Manhattan Study, Vol. I.,* McGraw-Hill, New York, 1962.

7 Coleman, J. V. The Group Factor in Military Psychiatry, *Am. J. Orthopsychiatry,* Vol. XV, April, 1946.

8 Leighton, Alexander H. *Psychiatric Disorder Among the Yoruba.* Cornell Univ. Press, Ithaca, New York, 1963.

9 Eaton, J. W. and Weil, R. J. *Culture and Mental Disorders.* The Free Press, Glencoe, Ill., 1955.

THE DYNAMICS OF THE PSYCHOTHERAPEUTIC
RELATIONSHIP
Jerome D. Frank

1 See, for instance, Talcott Parsons, "Illness and the Role of the Physician: A Sociological Perspective," *Amer. J. Orthopsychiatry* (1951) 21:452–460. Sebastian DeGrazia gives a brilliant if biased analysis of cultural and other factors contributing to the psychotherapist's influence over his patients. *See* DeGrazia, *Errors of Psychotherapy;* New York, Doubleday, 1952.

2 Norman Reider, "A Type of Transference to Institutions," *J. Hillside Hosp.* (1953) 2:23–29. For an interesting account of experimental studies on the context of a situation as an important determinant of influence see Robert R. Blake and Jane S. Mouton, "The Dynamics of Influence and Coercion," *Internat. J. Social Psychiatry* (1957) 2:263–274.

3 Sigmund Freud, *A General Introduction to Psychoanalysis;* New York, Liveright, 1920; p. 212.

4 Josef Breuer and Sigmund Freud, "Studies on Hysteria," in *The Complete Psychological Works* 2:3–305; London, Hogarth, 1955; p. 265.

5 Leslie Schaffer and Jerome K. Myers, "Psychotherapy and Social Stratification," PSYCHIATRY (1954) 17:83–93.

6 John C. Whitehorn and Barbara J. Betz, "A Study of Psychotherapeutic Relationships between Physicians and Schizophrenic Patients," *Amer. J. Psychiatry* (1954) 111:321–331.

7 *See,* for instance, George Winokur, " 'Brainwashing'—A Social Phenomenon of Our Time," *Hum. Organization* (1955) 13:16–18 and

Frederick Wyatt, "Climate of Opinion and Methods of Readjustment," *Amer. Psychologist* (1956) 11:537–542.

[8] Edward Glover, "Research Methods in Psycho-Analysis," *Internat. J. Psycho-Anal.* (1952) 33:403–409.

[9] Werner Wolff, "Fact and Value in Psychotherapy," *Amer. J. Psychotherapy* (1954) 8:466–486.

[10] Kenneth E. Appel, William T. Lhamon, J. Martin Myers, and William A. Harvey, "Long Term Psychotherapy," *Research Publ. Assn. N. and M. Disease* (1951) 31:21–34.

[11] See footnote 9; p. 470.

[12] Henri Ellenberger, "The Ancestry of Dynamic Psychotherapy," *Bull. Menninger Clin.* (1956) 20:288–299; p. 290.

[13] Jerome D. Frank, Lester H. Gliedman, Stanley D. Imber, Earl H. Nash, Jr., and Anthony R. Stone, "Why Patients Leave Psychotherapy," *AMA Arch. Neurol. and Psychiat.* (1957) 77:283–299. The results mentioned are reported in more detail in Imber, Frank, Gliedman, Nash, and Stone, "Suggestibility, Social Class and the Acceptance of Psychotherapy," *J. Clinical Psychol.* (1956) 12:341–344, and Imber, Nash and Stone, "Social Class and Duration of Psychotherapy," *J. Clinical Psychol.* (1955) 11: 281–284.

[14] See footnote 5.

[15] Frank and others, footnote 13; p. 294.

[16] With psychotics the suggested relation between degree of distress and willingness to trust the therapist often does not hold, because their distrust of others, especially those who seem to be offering help, is so profound. With such patients, the common core of successful psychotherapy may be the ability to break through this attitude and establish a trusting, confidential relationship. See, for example, John C. Whitehorn and Barbara J. Betz, "A Comparison of Psychotherapeutic Relationships between Physicians and Schizophrenic Patients When Insulin is Combined with Psychotherapy and When Psychotherapy Is Used Alone," *Amer. J. Psychiatry* (1957) 113:901–910. This common feature may explain the equally good results claimed by advocates of apparently incompatible therapeutic approaches. See, for example, *Psychotherapy with Schizophrenics*, edited by Eugene B. Brody and Fredrick C. Redlich; New York, Internat. Universities Press, 1952.

[17] See footnote 9.

[18] This point is interestingly discussed by B. F. Skinner in Carl R. Rogers and B. F. Skinner, "Some Issues Concerning the Control of Human Behavior: A Symposium," *Science* (1956) 124:1057–1066.

[19] The description of brainwashing in this paper is based on: L. E. Hinkle, Jr., and H. G. Wolff, "Communist Interrogation and Indoctrination of 'Enemies of the State,' " *AMA Arch. Neurol. and Psychiat.* (1956) 76:115–174; Robert J. Lifton, " 'Thought Reform' of Western Civilians in Chinese Communist Prisons," PSYCHIATRY (1956) 19:173–195; Lifton, "Chinese Communist Thought Reform," pp. 219–312; in *Group Processes: Transactions of the Third Conference*; New York, Josiah Macy, Jr. Foundation, 1957; Edgar H. Schein, "The Chinese Indoctrination Program for Prisoners of War," PSYCHIATRY (1956)

19:149–172. See also W. Sargant, *Battle for the Mind*; New York, Doubleday, 1957. He suggests that thought reform, religious revivals, and certain psychiatric treatments facilitate attitude change by producing excessive excitation, leading to emotional exhaustion and hypersuggestibility.

20 This reinforcement of certain of the prisoner's responses is analogous to operant conditioning, as will be discussed more fully below, in connection with psychotherapy.

21 Schein, footnote 19; p. 163, and footnote.

22 Schein, footnote 19; pp. 162–163.

23 Lifton, *Group Processes*, footnote 19; p. 269.

24 See footnote 19; p. 171.

25 Erving Goffman, "Interpersonal Persuasion," pp. 117–193; in *Group Processes: Transactions of the Third Conference*; New York, Josiah Macy, Jr. Foundation, 1957.

26 Lawrence S. Kubie, *Practical Aspects of Psychoanalysis*; New York, Norton, 1936; p. 140.

27 See footnote 26; p. 145.

28 Freud, footnote 3; pp. 319, 321 (Freud's italics).

29 Albert Stunkard, "Some Interpersonal Aspects of an Oriental Religion," PSYCHIATRY (1951) 14:419–431.

30 Hadley Cantril, *The Psychology of Social Movements*; New York, Wiley, 1941.

31 Edward S. Bordin, "Ambiguity as a Therapeutic Variable," *J. Consulting Psychology* (1955) 19:9–15.

32 For a brilliant analysis of compliance, identification and internalization in the influencing process see Herbert C. Kelman, "Compliance, Identification and Internalization: Three Processes of Attitude Change," *J. Conflict Resolution* (1958) 2:51–60.

33 Ernest R. Hilgard, *Theories of Learning*; New York, Appleton-Century-Crofts, 1948; Ch. 4, pp. 82–120.

34 Jurgen Ruesch, "Psychotherapy and Communication," pp. 180–187; in *Progress in Psychotherapy, 1956*, edited by Frieda Fromm-Reichmann and J. L. Moreno; New York, Grune and Stratton, 1956; p. 183.

35 Joel Greenspoon, "The Reinforcing Effect of Two Spoken Sounds on the Frequency of Two Responses," *Amer. J. Psychology* (1955) 68:409–416.

36 Kurt Salzinger and Stephanie Pisoni, "Reinforcement of Affect Responses of Schizophrenics During the Clinical Interview," *J. Abnormal and Social Psychol.* (1958) 57:84–90.

37 Edward J. Murray, "A Content-Analysis Method for Studying Psychotherapy," *Psychological Monographs* (1956) 70, Whole No. 420. The "Herbert Bryan" protocol is in Carl R. Rogers, *Counseling and Psychotherapy*; New York, Houghton Mifflin, 1942; pp. 259–437.

38 See, for instance, Kubie, footnote 26; Ch. 7.

39 Breuer and Freud, footnote 4; p. 295.

40 See Glover, footnote 8; p. 405, and "The Therapeutic Effect of Inexact Interpretation: A Contribution to the Theory of Suggestion,"

Internat. J. Psycho-Anal. (1931) 12:397–411. Other psychoanalytic writers have stressed the "hypersuggestibility" of the patient in analysis, seeing in the transference an analogy to hypnotic rapport. *See*, for example, Ida Macalpine, "The Development of the Transference," *Psychoanalytic Quart.* (1950) 19:501–539; Herman Nunberg, "Transference and Reality," *Internat. J. Psycho-Anal.* (1951) 32:1–9; C. Fisher, "Studies on the Nature of Suggestion: Pt. 1, Experimental Induction of Dreams by Direct Suggestion," *J. Amer. Psychoanal. Assn.* (1953) 1:222–255.

41 Rogers, footnote 18; p. 1063.

42 Wilhelm Stekel, *Interpretation of Dreams*; New York, Liveright, 1943, quoted by Werner Wolff in "Fact and Value in Psychotherapy," *Amer. J. Psychotherapy* (1954) 8:466–486; p. 466.

43 Carl R. Rogers, "A Research Program in Client-Centered Therapy," *Research Publ. Assn. N. and M. Disease* (1951) 31:106–113.

44 Murray, footnote 37.

45 Ralph W. Heine, "A Comparison of Patients' Reports on Psychotherapeutic Experience with Psychoanalytic, Nondirective and Adlerian Therapists," *Amer. J. Psychotherapy* (1953) 7:16–23.

46 David Rosenthal, "Changes in Some Moral Values Following Psychotherapy," *J. Consulting Psychol.* (1955) 19:431–436. For historical examples of "doctrinal compliance" see Jan Ehrenwald, "The Telepathy Hypothesis and Doctrinal Compliance in Psychotherapy," *Amer. J. Psychotherapy* (1957) 11:359–379.

47 For example, in an experimental study of psychotherapy with a schizophrenic, M. B. Parloff found that ". . . although topic choice appeared to follow the therapist's values remarkably closely, the patient's own evaluation of these topics in some instances, moved quite independently. . . . This finding suggests that the patient may be superficially compliant to the unconsciously expressed expectations of the therapist, without, however, internalizing such values." M. B. Parloff, "Communication of Values and Therapeutic Change," paper read at the American Psychological Association meeting, New York, 1957.

48 Bruno Bettelheim, "Remarks on the Psychological Appeal of Totalitarianism," *Amer. J. Economics and Sociology* (1952) 12:89–96. Recent experimental studies have found that inducing a person to speak overtly in favor of some position changes his private opinion in the direction of the one he had publicly stated. See Irving L. Janis and Bert T. King, "The Influence of Role-Playing on Opinion Change," *J. Abnormal and Social Psychol.* (1954) 49:211–218; Bert T. King and Irving L. Janis, "Comparison of the Effectiveness of Improvised Versus Non-Improvised Role-Playing in Producing Opinion Changes," *Hum. Relations* (1956) 9:177–186.

49 W. S. Verplanck, "The Operant Conditioning of Human Motor Behavior," *Psychological Bull.* (1956) 53:70–83.

50 Morris B. Parloff, Herbert C. Kelman, and Jerome D. Frank, "Comfort, Effectiveness, and Self-Awareness as Criteria of Improvement in Psychotherapy," *Amer. J. Psychiatry* (1954) 111:343–351.

51 See footnote 13. See also Rogers, footnote 43.

52 Clara Thompson, *Psychoanalysis: Evolution and Development*; New York, Hermitage House, 1950; p. 235.

53 J. Seeman, quoted in J. M. Schlien, "Time-Limited Psychotherapy: An Experimental Investigation of Practical Values and Theoretical Implications," *J. Counseling Psychol.* (1957) 4:318–322.

54 See, for instance, Jacob H. Conn, "Brief Psychotherapy of the Sex Offender: A Report of a Liaison Service Between a Court and a Private Psychiatrist," *J. Clinical Psychopathol.* (1949) 10:1–26; Jacob H. Conn, "Hypnosynthesis III: Hypnotherapy of Chronic War Neuroses with a Discussion of the Value of Abreaction, Regression, and Revivication," *J. Clinical and Experimental Hypnosis* (1953) 1:29–43.

55 John N. Fortin and D. W. Abse, "Group Psychotherapy with Peptic Ulcer," *Internat. J. Group Psychotherapy* (1956) 6:383–391; p. 385.

56 Fortin and Abse, footnote 55; p. 390 and following.

57 M. N. Chappell, J. J. Stefano, J. S. Rogerson, and F. H. Pike, "The Value of Group Psychological Procedures in the Treatment of Peptic Ulcer," *Amer. J. Digestive Diseases and Nutrition* (1937) 3:813–817.

58 One patient could not be located.

59 Unfortunately Fortin and Abse do not state how many of their patients had mild recurrences, and Chappell and his colleagues do not give the improvement rate at the end of a year, so the results of the two treatment programs cannot be strictly compared. Assuming that the student who hemorrhaged in the first study is equivalent to the "relapsed" patients in the second, Chappell had the same recurrence rate at the end of three years that Fortin and Abse had at the end of a year—about 10 percent in each series. On the unlikely assumption that the 4 patients lost to the Chappell study had relapsed, their three-year recurrence rate is about 20 percent. Including the mild recurrences this brings the Chappell three-year relapse rate to about 50 percent. Even this figure is well below the expected recurrence rate of over 75 percent mentioned by Fortin and Abse.

60 Jerome D. Frank, Lester H. Gliedman, Stanley D. Imber, Anthony R. Stone, and Earl H. Nash, Jr., "Patients' Expectancies and Relearning as Factors Determining Improvement in Psychotherapy," *Amer. J. Psychiatry*, in press.

61 J. M. Schlien, "An Experimental Investigation of Time Limited, Client Centered Therapy," University of Chicago Counselling Center Discussion, Papers, Vol. 2, 1956. According to Schlien (see footnote 53), patients on time limited therapy showed changes on TAT scores in the follow-up period which were interpreted as undesirable, despite their maintained improvement on the other indices. The sources of this discrepancy are now under study.

62 Franz Alexander, "Discussion of 'Aims and Limitations of Psychotherapy' by Paul H. Hoch," pp. 82–86; in Fromm-Reichmann and Moreno, footnote 34; p. 82.

63 For interesting biographical vignettes of nine such converts, see H. Begbie, *Twice-Born Men*; London, Revell, 1909.

64 Benjamin Weininger, "The Interpersonal Factor in the Religious Experience," *Psychoanalysis* (1955) 3:27–44.

65 William James, *The Varieties of Religious Experience*; New York, The Modern Library, 1936; p. 200.

66 Pierre Janet's discussion of "Miraculous Healing," Ch. 1 in *Psychological Healing*, Vol. 1 (New York, Macmillan, 1925) is the best account of miracle cures which has come to my attention. A very good recent account is found in Ruth Cranston, *The Miracle of Lourdes*; New York, McGraw-Hill, 1955.

67 H. Rehder, "Wunderheilungen, Ein Experiment," *Hippokrates* (1955) 26:577–580.

68 Janet, footnote 66; p. 48.

69 H. Wolff, "What Hopes Does for Man," *Saturday Review of Literature*, January 8, 1957; p. 45.

70 A. A. Kurland, "The Drug Placebo—Its Psychodynamic and Conditional Reflex Action," *Behavioral Science* (1957) 2:101–110, offers a recent survey of knowledge as to the effects of placebos.

71 B. Bloch, "Ueber die Heilung der Warzen durch Suggestion," *Klin. Wochenschr.* (1927) 6:2271–2325.

72 F. A. Volgyesi, " 'School for Patients,' Hypnosis-Therapy and Psycho-Prophylaxis," *British J. Medical Hypnotism* (1954) 5:8–17.

73 J. L. Hampson, David Rosenthal, and Jerome D. Frank, "A Comparative Study of the Effect of Mephenesin and Placebo on the Symptomatology of a Mixed Group of Psychiatric Outpatients," *Bull. Johns Hopkins Hosp.* (1954) 95:170–177.

74 Appel and others; see footnote 10.

75 See footnote 6.

76 David Rosenthal and Jerome D. Frank, "Psychotherapy and the Placebo Effect," *Psychological Bull.* (1956) 53:294–302. See also the editorial by J. C. Whitehorn, "Psychiatric Implications of the 'Placebo Effect,' " *Amer. J. Psychiatry* (1958) 114:662–664.

77 Lester H. Gliedman, Earl H. Nash, Anthony R. Stone, and Jerome D. Frank, "Reduction of Symptoms by Pharmacologically Inert Substances and by Short Term Psychotherapy," *AMA Arch. Neurol. and Psychiat.* (1958) 79:345–351.

78 L. Lasagna, F. Mosteller, J. M. von Felsinger, and H. K. Beecher, "A Study of the Placebo Response," *Amer. J. Medicine* (1954) 16:770–779.

79 See, for example, the contributions to *Progress in Psychotherapy, 1956*, footnote 34.

80 Frank, and others, footnote 13.

81 M. Balint, "The Doctor, His Patient, and the Illness," *Lancet* (1955) 268:683–688.

82 Walter Modell, *The Relief of Symptoms*; Philadelphia, Saunders, 1955; p. 56.

83 Sydney G. Margolin advocates deliberately fostering regression of certain patients in "On Some Principles of Therapy," *Amer. J. Psychiatry* (1958) 114:1087–1096.

[84] Jerome D. Frank, "Psychotherapeutic Aspects of Symptomatic Treatment," *Amer. J. Psychiatry* (1946) 103:21–25.

[85] Sandor Rado sees as one of the critical tasks in the treatment of behavior disorders, "to generate in [the patient] an emotional matrix dominated by the welfare emotions [pleasurable desire, joy, affection, love, self-respect and pride]"; see *Psychoanalysis of Behavior*; New York, Grune and Stratton, 1956; p. 253. Perhaps faith should be included in the list.

[86] For a penetrating discussion of this issue, see Ernst Kris, "Psychoanalytic Propositions," Ch. 22, pp. 332–351; in *Psychological Theory*, edited by M. H. Marx; New York, Macmillan, 1951.

INSTITUTIONALISM IN MENTAL HOSPITALS
J. K. Wing

REFERENCES

Belknap, I. (1956). *Human Problems of a State Mental Hospital.* New York: McGraw Hill.

Bettelheim, B., & Sylvester, E. (1948). A therapeutic milieu. *Amer. J. Orthopsychiat.* 18, 191–206.

Brooke, E. (1957). A national study of schizophrenic patients in relation to occupation. *Int. Congr. Psychiat.* III, 52–63.

Brown, G. W. (1960a). Social factors influencing length of hospital stay of schizophrenic patients. *Brit. med. J.* 2, 1300–1302.

Brown, G. W. (1960b). Length of hospital stay and schizophrenia: A review of statistical studies. *Acta Psychiat.* 35, 414–430.

Carstairs, G. M., & Wing, J. K. (1958). Attitudes of the general public to mental illness. *Brit. med. J.* 2, 594–597.

Caudill, W. (1958). *The Psychiatric Hospital as a Small Society.* Cambridge, Mass.: Harvard University Press.

Early, D. F. (1960). The Industrial Therapy Organisation (Bristol): A development of work in hospital. *Lancet,* 2, 754–757.

Ellenberger, H. F. (1960). Zoological garden and mental hospital. *Canad. Psychiat. Ass. J.* 5, 136–149.

Fish, F. J. (1957). The classification of schizophrenia. The views of Kleist and his co-workers. *J. ment. Sci.* 103, 443–463.

Fish, F. J. (1958). Leonhard's classification of schizophrenia. *J. ment. Sci.* 104, 943–971.

Goffman, E. (1958). The characteristics of total institutions. In *Symposium on Prev. and Soc. Psychiatry,* Washington, 1958. Walter Reed Army Institute of Research.

Goffman, E. (1959). The moral career of the mental patients. *Psychiatry,* 22, 123–142.

Kety, S. S. (1959). Biochemical theories of schizophrenia. *Science,* 129, 1528–1532.

Kramer, M., Goldstein, H., Israel, R. H. & Johnson, N. A. (1955). A historical study of the disposition of first admissions to a state

324

mental hospital. *Public Health Monographs* No. 32, U.S. Public Health Service, Washington.

Leonhard, K. (1957). *Die Aufteilung der endogenen Psychosen.* Berlin. Akademie Verlag.

Lewis, A. J. (1953). Health as a social concept. *Brit. J. Sociol.* 5, 109–124.

Merton, R. K. (1957). *Social Theory and Social Structure.* Glencoe, Ill.: The Free Press.

Norris, V. (1956). A statistical study of the influence of marriage on the hospital care of the mentally sick. *J. ment. Sci.* 102, 467–486.

Schein, E. H. (1956). The Chinese indoctrination program for prisoners of war. *Psychiatry,* 19, 149–172.

Scott, P. (1960). The treatment of psychopaths. *Brit. med. J.* 1, 1641–1645.

Sommer, R. (1959). Patients who grow old in a mental hospital. *Geriatrics,* 14, 581–590.

Titmuss, R. M. (1958). The hospital and its patients. In *Essays on the Welfare State.* London. Allen & Unwin.

Titmuss, R. M. (1959). Community care as a challenge. *The Times,* 12 May.

Wing, J. K. (1960a). The measurement of behaviour in chronic schizophrenia. *Acta Psychiat.* 35, 245–254.

Wing, J. K. (1960b). A pilot experiment in the rehabilitation of long hospitalised schizophrenic patients. *Brit. J. prev. soc. Med.* 14, 173–180.

Wing, J. K. (1961). A simple and reliable subclassification of chronic schizophrenia. *J. ment. Sc.,* in press.

Wootton, B. (1959). *Social Science and Social Pathology.* London: Allen & Unwin.

THE MYTH OF MENTAL ILLNESS
Thomas S. Szasz

[1] Freud went so far as to say that: "I consider ethics to be taken for granted. Actually I have never done a mean thing" (Jones, 1957, p. 247). This surely is a strange thing to say for someone who has studied man as a social being as closely as did Freud. I mention it here to show how the notion of "illness" (in the case of psychoanalysis, "psychopathology," or "mental illness") was used by Freud—and by most of his followers—as a means for classifying certain forms of human behavior as falling within the scope of medicine, and hence (by *fiat*) outside that of ethics!

REFERENCES

Hollingshead, A. B., & Redlich, F. C. *Social class and mental illness.* New York: Wiley, 1958.

Jones, E. *The life and work of Sigmund Freud.* Vol. III. New York: Basic Books, 1957.

Langer, S. K. *Philosophy in a new key*. New York: Mentor Books, 1953.

Peters, R. S. *The concept of motivation*. London: Routledge & Kegan Paul, 1958.

Szasz, T. S. Malingering: "Diagnosis" or social condemnation? *AMA Arch. Neurol. Psychiat.*, 1956, 76, 432–443.

Szasz, T. S. *Pain and pleasure: A study of bodily feelings*. New York: Basic Books, 1957. (a)

Szasz, T. S. The problem of psychiatric nosology: A contribution to a situational analysis of psychiatric operations. *Amer. J. Psychiat.*, 1957, 114, 405–413. (b)

Szasz, T. S. On the theory of psychoanalytic treatment. *Int. J. Psycho-Anal.*, 1957, 38, 166–182. (c)

Szasz, T. S. Psychiatry, ethics and the criminal law. *Columbia Law Rev.*, 1958, 58, 183–198.

Szasz, T. S. Moral conflict and psychiatry, *Yale Rev.*, 1959, in press.

PERSONALITY DISORDER *IS* DISEASE
David P. Ausubel

REFERENCES

Ausubel, D. P. *Ego development and the personality disorders*. New York: Grune & Stratton, 1952.

Ausubel, D. P. Relationships between psychology and psychiatry: The hidden issues. *Amer. Psychologist*, 1956, 11, 99–105.

Dreyfuss, F., & Czaczkes, J. W. Blood cholesterol and uric acid of healthy medical students under the stress of an examination. *AMA Arch. intern. Med.*, 1959, 103, 708.

Mowrer, O. H. "Sin," the lesser of two evils. *Amer. Psychologist*, 1960, 15, 301–304.

Szasz, T. S. The myth of mental illness. *Amer. Psychologist*, 1960, 15, 113–118.

PARANOIA AND THE DYNAMICS OF EXCLUSION
Edwin M. Lemert

[1] In a subsequent article Cameron (2) modified his original conception, but not of the social aspects of paranoia, which mainly concern us.

[2] The interaction in some ways is similar to that used with children, particularly the *"enfant terrible."* The function of language in such interaction was studied by Sapir[16] years ago.

[3] For a systematic analysis of the organizational difficulties in removing an "unpromotable" person from a position see (9).

[4] One of the cases in the first study.

[5] This technique in even more systematic form is sometimes used in protecting the President of the United States in "White House cases."

REFERENCES

1. Cameron, N., "The Paranoid Pseudocommunity," *American Journal of Sociology*, 1943, 46, 33–38.

2. Cameron, N., "The Paranoid Pseudocommunity Revisited," *American Journal of Sociology*, 1959, 65, 52–58.

3. Cumming, E., and J. Cumming, *Closed Ranks*, Cambridge, Mass.: Harvard Press, 1957, Ch. VI.

4. Dentler, R. A., and K. T. Erikson, "The Functions of Deviance in Groups," *Social Problems*, 1959, 7, 102.

5. Goffman, E., "The Moral Career of the Mental Patient," *Psychiatry*, 1959, 22, 127 ff.

6. Jaco, E. G., "Attitudes Toward, and Incidence of Mental Disorder: A Research Note," *Southwestern Social Science Quarterly*, June, 1957, p. 34.

7. Kine, F. F., "Aliens' Paranoid Reaction," *Journal of Mental Science*, 1951, 98, 589–594.

8. Lemert, E., "Legal Commitment and Social Control," *Sociology and Social Research*, 1946, 30, 33–338.

9. Levenson, B., "Bureaucratic Succession," in *Complex Organizations*, A. Etzioni, (ed.), New York: Holt, Rinehart and Winston, 1961, 362–395.

10. Listivan, I., "Paranoid States: Social and Cultural Aspects," *Medical Journal of Australia*, 1956, 776–778.

11. Loomis, J. L., "Communications, The Development of Trust, and Cooperative Behavior," *Human Relations*, 1959, 12, 305–315.

12. Marmor, J., "Science, Health and Group Opposition" (mimeographed paper), 1958.

13. Milner, K. O., "The Environment as a Factor in the Etiology of Criminal Paranoia," *Journal of Mental Science*, 1949, 95, 124–132.

14. Ödegard, Ö., "A Clinical Study of Delayed Admissions to a Mental Hospital," *Mental Hygiene*, 1958, 42, 66–77.

15. Pederson, S., "Psychological Reactions to Extreme Social Displacement (Refugee Neuroses)," *Psychoanalytic Review*, 1946, 36, 344–354.

16. Sapir, E., "Abnormal Types of Speech in Nootka," *Canada Department of Mines*, Memoir 62, 1915, No. 5.

17. Stanton, A. H., and M. S. Schwartz, *The Mental Hospital*, New York: Basic Books, 1954, 200–210.

18. Tyhurst, J. S., "Paranoid Patterns," in A. H. Leighton, J. A. Clausen, and R. Wilson (eds.), *Exploration in Social Psychiatry*, New York: Basic Books, 1957, Ch. II.

NOTES ON THE SOCIOLOGY OF DEVIANCE
Kai T. Erikson

[1] Emile Durkheim, *The Rules of Sociological Method* (translated by S. A. Solovay and J. H. Mueller), New York: The Free Press, 1958.

2 The best known statements of this general position, of course, are by Robert K. Merton and Talcott Parsons. Merton, *Social Theory and Social Structures* (revised edition), New York: The Free Press, 1957; and Parsons, *The Social System*, New York: The Free Press, 1951.

3 Daniel Glaser and Kent Rice, "Crime, Age, and Employment," *American Sociological Review*, 24 (1959), pp. 679–86.

4 Emile Durkheim, *The Division of Labor in Society* (translated by George Simpson), New York: The Free Press, 1952. See particularly Chapter 2, Book 1.

5 Emile Durkheim, *The Rules of Sociological Method, op. cit.*

6 Talcott Parsons, *The Social System, op. cit.*

7 For a good description of this process in the modern prison, *see* Gresham Sykes, *The Society of Captives*, Princeton: Princeton University Press, 1958. For views of two different types of mental hospital settings, see Erving Goffman, "The Characteristics of Total Institutions," *Symposium on Preventive and Social Psychiatry*, Washington, D.C.: Walter Reed Army Institute of Research, 1957; and Kai T. Erikson, "Patient Role and Social Uncertainty: A Dilemma of the Mentally Ill," *Psychiatry*, 20 (1957), pp. 263–74.

8 Talcott Parsons, *op. cit.*, has given the classical description of how this role transfer works in the case of medical patients.

9 Harold Garfinkel, "Successful Degradation Ceremonies," *American Journal of Sociology*, 61 (1956), pp. 420–24.

10 Albert K. Cohen, for example, speaking for most sociologists, seems to take the question for granted: "It would seem that the control of deviant behavior is, by definition, a culture goal." In "The Study of Social Disorganization and Deviant Behavior," Merton et al., editors, *Sociology Today*. New York: Basic Books, 1959, p. 465.

11 Georg Simmel, *Conflict* (translated by Kurt H. Wolff), New York: The Free Press, 1955, pp. 15–16.

Index